SpringerBriefs in Public Health

SpringerBriefs in Public Health present concise summaries of cutting-edge research and practical applications from across the entire field of public health, with contributions from medicine, bioethics, health economics, public policy, biostatistics, and sociology.

The focus of the series is to highlight current topics in public health of interest to a global audience, including health care policy; social determinants of health; health issues in developing countries; new research methods; chronic and infectious disease epidemics; and innovative health interventions.

Featuring compact volumes of 50 to 125 pages, the series covers a range of content from professional to academic. Possible volumes in the series may consist of timely reports of state-of-the art analytical techniques, reports from the field, snapshots of hot and/or emerging topics, elaborated theses, literature reviews, and in-depth case studies. Both solicited and unsolicited manuscripts are considered for publication in this series.

Briefs are published as part of Springer's eBook collection, with millions of users worldwide. In addition, Briefs are available for individual print and electronic purchase.

Briefs are characterized by fast, global electronic dissemination, standard publishing contracts, easy-to-use manuscript preparation and formatting guidelines, and expedited production schedules. We aim for publication 8-12 weeks after acceptance.

More information about this series at http://www.springer.com/series/10138

Sima Barmania • Michael J. Reiss

Islam and Health Policies Related to HIV Prevention in Malaysia

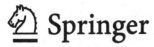 Springer

Sima Barmania
UCL Institute of Education
University College London
London, United Kingdom

Michael J. Reiss
UCL Institute of Education
University College London
London, United Kingdom

ISSN 2192-3698   ISSN 2192-3701   (electronic)
SpringerBriefs in Public Health
ISBN 978-3-319-68908-1   ISBN 978-3-319-68909-8   (eBook)
https://doi.org/10.1007/978-3-319-68909-8

Library of Congress Control Number: 2017954581

Printed on acid-free paper

This Springer imprint is published by Springer Nature
The registered company is Springer International Publishing AG
The registered company address is: Gewerbestrasse 11, 6330 Cham, Switzerland

*Dedicated to Olima, Hansa Patel-Kanwal,
and Hiroko Hirose*

Acknowledgements

The authors would like to acknowledge PT Foundation, JAKIM, Malaysian Ministry of Health, United Nations University—International Institute for Global Health, National University of Malaysia, UKM Research ethics committee, and Prof. Syed Aljunid.

Contents

About the Authors

Sima Barmania, BMedSci, MBBS, MPH, PhD, is a British medical doctor in global health, based in London, United Kingdom, and Kuala Lumpur, Malaysia. She is a freelance writer, consultant, and an honorary research associate at UCL Institute of Education in London, UK. She qualified in medicine from Queen Mary University of London with an intercalated degree in community health sciences and undertook her Master's in Public Health from London School of Hygiene and Tropical Medicine. She completed her PhD in 2016 at United Nations University—Institute for Global Health, in collaboration with the National University of Malaysia, where her doctoral research explored the role of Islam in shaping HIV prevention in Malaysia. She is interested in the interface between public health, religion, and culture as well as broader interests spanning reproductive and mental health, and public health advocacy. Having had a long-running blog in the *Independent*, she also writes freelance for *The Lancet* medical journal and other media outlets. Her interests also include spirituality, world religions, interfaith and peace education.

Michael J. Reiss, MBA, PGCE, PhD, is professor of Science Education at UCL Institute of Education in London, United Kingdom; visiting professor at the Universities of Kiel, Leeds, and York and the Royal Veterinary College; honorary fellow of the British Science Association and of the College of Teachers; docent at the University of Helsinki in Finland; and a fellow of the Academy of Social Sciences.

A former director of Education at the Royal Society, the inaugural editor of the academic journal *Sex Education*, and former specialist adviser to the House of Commons Education Committee PSHE (Personal, Social and Health Education) Inquiry, he is also a priest in the Church of England and president of the International Society for Science and Religion. His research and consultancy interests are in science education, bioethics, and sex education.

Books of his include: Abrahams, I. & Reiss, M. J. (Eds) (2017) *Enhancing Learning with Effective Practical Science 11-16*, Bloomsbury; Reiss, M. J. & White, J. (2013) *An Aims-based Curriculum*, IOE Press; Jones, A., McKim, A. & Reiss, M.

(Eds) (2010) *Ethics in the Science and Technology Classroom: A New Approach to Teaching and Learning*, Sense; Jones, L. & Reiss, M. J. (Eds) (2007) *Teaching about Scientific Origins: Taking Account of Creationism*, Peter Lang; Braund, M. & Reiss, M. J. (Eds) (2004) *Learning Science Outside the Classroom*, RoutledgeFalmer; Levinson, R. & Reiss, M. J. (Eds) (2003) *Key Issues in Bioethics: A Guide for Teachers*, RoutledgeFalmer; Halstead, J. M. & Reiss, M. J. (2003) *Values in Sex Education: From Principles to Practice*, RoutledgeFalmer; Reiss, M. J. (2000) *Understanding Science Lessons: Five Years of Science Teaching*, Open University Press; Chapman, J. L. & Reiss, M. J. (1999). *Ecology: Principles and Applications*, Cambridge University Press; Reiss, M. J. & Mabud, S. A. (Eds) (1998) *Sex Education and Religion*, The Islamic Academy; Reiss, M. J. & Straughan, R. (1996). *Improving Nature? The Science and Ethics of Genetic Engineering*, Cambridge University Press; Reiss, M. J. (1993) *Science Education for a Pluralist Society*, Open University Press; King, A. & Reiss, M. J. (Eds) (1993) *The Multicultural Dimension of the National Curriculum*, Falmer Press; and Reiss, M. J. (1989) *The Allometry of Growth and Reproduction*, Cambridge University Press.

Chapter 1
Introduction

Religion, Health and Society

There is perhaps no more divisive a topic than that of the subject of religion (Dawkins 2006; Armstrong 1993). Some people vehemently believe that religion is the source of all conflict and has left few positive impressions over the centuries; rather it has produced a legacy of war, fanaticism, hypocrisy and condemnation. Others, with equal fervour, deem religion to be the only source of salvation and peace, central to the way they live their lives and conduct themselves. However, even if one is ambivalent about religion, the chances are high that religion influences one's life as many of the current cultural norms and laws are based on religion, at least to some degree. This is true both for Eastern and Western societies, whether it is as simple as religious holidays in the calendar year which result in a welcome public holiday or many of the phrases used even in contemporary language. For those who have a greater affiliation with a particular religion, this may infiltrate to every aspect of their lives, from what they eat and what they wear to whom they chose as their spouse. Furthermore, the distinction between 'religious' and 'irreligious' is not always one that can be tightly drawn, as many who deem themselves as 'irreligious' follow certain religious-derived practices, while those who are 'religious' may equally ignore certain features of their religion.

Religion often plays a central role in people's health and for some this starts even before an individual has the ability to cogitate on their belief system. For example, both Muslims and Jews chose circumcision for the newborn male child, a decision made by the parents on behalf of a child who is too young to consent. Male circumcision in Judaism has been performed for centuries, with little clear physical benefit or reasoning other than the religious one of a mark of the covenant between God and his people. Interestingly, in recent years there has been scientific evidence that male circumcision offers benefits for health as a child (treatment for paraphimosis and personal hygiene) and also some protection as an adult to Human Immunodeficiency

© The Author(s) 2018
S. Barmania, M.J. Reiss, *Islam and Health Policies Related
to HIV Prevention in Malaysia*, SpringerBriefs in Public Health,
https://doi.org/10.1007/978-3-319-68909-8_1

Virus (HIV) transmission, so much so that male circumcision has been rolled out in parts of Africa as a contribution to HIV prevention. Thus, something that was once reserved for a particular religious tribe has now become a credible medical and public health practice. On a day-to-day level, religion often influences individual health behaviours in ways that can either be positive or negative, for example religious fasting, use of alcohol and drugs (both medicinal and illicit) and sexual practices (Koenig 2008). Notwithstanding these points, the role of religion transcends its impact on physical health; religion can often be a strong empowering coping mechanism and can provide a social structure for dealing with stress and ill health or act as a catalyst for a fatalistic lack of responsibility for one's health.

If one subscribes to the longstanding and well-known World Health Organisation (WHO) definition of health: 'Health is a state of complete physical, mental and social well-being and not merely the absence of disease or infirmity' (WHO 1948), religion can then be argued to have a significant influence on health and well-being. Indeed, religion can then be seen as a determinant of health, just like (other aspects of) culture, even if only somewhat peripherally. However, in the Western World, health is often considered within a predominantly secular environment with little discussion around the interplay of religion and health. Although public health models do take into consideration the influence of culture (Dahlgren and Whitehead 1992), there has been surprisingly little discussion of the impact of faith and religion on health.

Although, in theory, many religious traditions try to differentiate between culture and religion, in reality there is often great overlap. Until recently, there has been little acknowledgement of the contribution of faith and faith-based organisations to health but this stance may not only be counterproductive but obstructive. The absence of faith and religion in such discussions is in part due to negative connotations arising from the historical antecedents of religious imperialism, colonialism, proselytizing and hidden motivations. In addition, faith and religion are often seen to be contrary to modernity, and Tyndale argues that religion is almost seen as an 'antidevelopment force' (Tyndale 2003). Religion is often perceived as being divisive and faith seen as a major source of conflict in the world with politics often the catalyst. Many have highlighted the substantial negative contribution of religion; judgement and inclusive club mentality simply reinforce divisions that already exist in society (Flannigan 2010).

Aside from moral and ideological objections, faith-based groups are often seen as lacking in professionalism when they get involved with health matters, with little emphasis on evaluation, thus raising doubts about their effectiveness. Despite such assertions, religion matters and for reasons that range from service delivery to its effect on health promotion. Faith-based organisations make a substantial contribution to health services in the developing world, with attempts to quantify this suggesting a figure of around 50% (Obaid 2005). In some regions faith-based groups are often the sole source of support and often arose out of need. Religion can often drive health policy, as in the case of the United States President Emergency Plan for AIDS Relief (PEPFAR) and 'Abstinence, Be faithful and Condom' (ABC) campaigns and can undermine implementation of public health programmes if such programmes fail to take religion into account.

However, there are a plethora of valuable assets in the religion-health field that can be tapped into to the advantage of health measures; in general, assets located in or held by a religious entity can be leveraged for the purposes of development or public health (African Religious Health Assets Programme 2007). These can be either 'tangible' including facilities, such as places of worship, or intangible', such as motivation and mobilizing capacities that are rooted in various dimensions of religious faith, whilst religious leaders often have a great wealth of local knowledge and networks. And finally, on the far end of the intangible spectrum, are assets of compassion, forgiveness, social capital and hope. This is especially true in many developing countries and when looking at global health, where health is set amidst a backdrop of strong religious affiliations. Historically, there was a marked institutional and organisational shift in attention to the role of faith and an awareness that partnerships with Faith-Based Organisations (FBOs) were required if the Millennium Development Goals were to be achieved (UNFPA 2008; UNAIDS 2009, 2010).

Religion and HIV

Often, the discrimination and taboos surrounding HIV are most acutely felt by those from a religious community, whilst these communities have often liked to distance themselves from any association with HIV. The interplay between religion and health in the HIV arena is often controversial (Haynes 2007). Religions have helped but also have hindered health progress by denying HIV's existence, moralising HIV, stigmatising and interfering with health promotion campaigns. There are some religious leaders who have even described Acquired Immune Deficiency Syndrome (AIDS) as the 'wrath of God' (Badri 1997). Over time there has been a welcome shift in appreciation of the fundamental role that religion plays in many societies and a realisation that many affected by HIV espouse strong religious convictions. In Muslim communities it is becoming increasingly acknowledged that the global burden of HIV is not simply limited to the non-Muslim population, but is an issue of the Muslim world as well. Marina Mahathir, former director of the Malaysian Aids Council (MAC), explains that although the prevalence of HIV in Muslim countries is relatively low in comparison with other regions, it is still a significant problem (Mahathir 2009).

HIV in the Muslim World

Unfortunately, it is difficult to ascertain the number of people living with HIV from a Muslim background as often there is a lack of reporting and even misinformation, while many epidemiological or surveillance studies do not include religion within their groupings. Muslim communities, like many others, have a strong tendency to ignore the existence of HIV, creating a culture of denial, and have typically responded with the familiar adage of 'not our problem', believing (or hoping) that being Muslim is a panacea to protect against HIV (Mahathir 2009). However, in reality, Muslim societies do not necessarily act in the accordance with the teachings of the Qur'an. Muslims engage in the same behaviours that fuel the transmission of HIV elsewhere, yet are reluctant to admit it (Kelley and Eberstadt 2005); what transpires is a separation of public morality and private reality. Such a separation does not avoid the problem but merely accelerates the epidemic by making HIV prevention strategies more difficult to implement. Some academics believe that the issue of HIV/AIDS in the Muslim world is a potential public health crisis (Kelley and Eberstadt 2005). Ultimately, although Muslims may endeavour to live by Islamic practices, in reality some Islamic rules such as male circumcision are assiduously adhered to whilst others, such as the prohibition on sex outside marriage, are not. Often in Islamic communities there is a strong emphasis on privacy, which relates to all spheres of life, including one's sexual conduct, distinct from the Western concept of greater openness. One Muslim country with a rising HIV prevalence is Malaysia, a country not traditionally associated with HIV, even though the first case of HIV was documented in the late 1980s.

Malaysia

There is often a misconception that HIV does not occur in countries that are predominantly Muslim, such as Malaysia. However, the reality is that HIV is of growing importance in Malaysia, yet often the response to HIV/AIDS has been surrounded in denial and taboo. HIV is often associated with practices that are highly sensitive and forbidden in Islam, such as sex outside marriage, which further adds to the stigma and discrimination of Malaysian People Living with HIV (PLHIV). Those groups which are likely to engage in sex before marriage are less likely to actively seek access to services that could prevent the transmission of HIV or to be tested for it. High risk groups, such as Men who have Sex with Men (MSM), Transgender Women and Sex Workers are more likely to retreat underground and not engage with prevention services, which constitutes a lost opportunity to prevent HIV amongst those at risk. Western secular HIV prevention models are far more open at engaging with such high risk groups but such models are not a particularly 'good fit'; in Malaysia as they are considered at odds with the teachings of Islam.

Although there is a growing amount of information and research related to HIV in Malaysia, there is very little relating to Islam and HIV, with a complete absence of any knowledge relating to how Islam affects HIV prevention policies in the country. There has been an urgent need to critically analyse how perceptions of Islam actually affect HIV prevention policy in Malaysia. Furthermore, such analysis needs to be undertaken from a neutral, public health perspective by those who are cognisant of and sensitive to the Islamic and political context. The study reported in this book is intended to contribute substantially to understanding regarding HIV amongst Muslims in Malaysia and the wider Muslim World, with a view to making concrete recommendations for policy and practice.

References

African Religious Health Assets Programme (ARHAP). (2007). *Appreciating assets: The contribution of religion to universal access in Africa*. South Africa: Cape Town.

Armstrong, K. (1993). *History of God*. London: Ballantine Books.

Badri, M. (1997). *The AIDS crisis: A natural product of modernity's sexual revolution*. Kuala Lumpur: International Institute of Islamic Thought and Civilisation.

Dahlgren, G., & Whitehead, M. (1992). *Layered influence on health*. New York: WHO.

Dawkins, R. (2006). *The God delusion*. London: Black Swan.

Flannigan, S. T. (2010). *For the love of God: NGOs and religious identity in a violent world*. Vermont: Kumarian Press.

Haynes, J. (2007). *Religion and development: Conflict or cooperation?* Basingstoke: Palgrave Macmillan.

Kelley, L. M., & Eberstadt, N. (2005). *Behind the veil of a public health crisis: HIV/AIDS in the Muslim world*. Washington: National Bureau of Asian Research.

Koenig, H. G. (2008). *Medicine, religion and health*. Pennsylvania: Templeton.

Mahathir, M. (2009). Fatal confluences? Islam, gender, and AIDS in Malaysia. In F. Esack & S. Chiddy (Eds.), *Islam and AIDS: Between scorn, pity and justice* (pp. 105–123). Oxford: One World.

Obaid, T. (2005). Religion and reproductive health and rights. *Journal of the American Academy of Religion, 73*(4), 1155–1173.

Tyndale, W. (2003). Idealism and practicality: The role of religion in development. *Journal of international Development, 46*(4), 22–28.

UNAIDS. (2009). *UNAIDS strategic framework: Partnership with faith based organisations*. Geneva: UNAIDS.

UNAIDS. (2010). *Religious leadership in response to HIV*. Geneva: UNAIDS.

UNFPA. (2008). *Culture matters: Lessons from a legacy of engaging with faith based organisations*. New York: UNFPA.

WHO. (1948). *Preamble to the constitution of the world health organisation as adopted by the International Health Conference*. New York: WHO.

Chapter 2
Background

Malaysia's Historical Context

Malaysia, a country in South East Asia, has a rich culture with a history over the past 100 years that shows it progressing from a colonised nation to one that has developed economically and now is democratically ruled. Malaysia, like a number of countries, was under British colonial rule and many critics have described the impact of colonialism on Muslim societies, both during the time of the empire and in the decades succeeding it. In discussing the effects of colonialism on the Muslim world, Fuller (2012) argues that imperial rule both distorted cultured traditions whilst at the same time the role of the imam was denigrated. Decolonization, although accompanied by a relinquishing of imperial power, hegemony and foreign rule on countries, still meant that external input occurred via organisations such as the World Bank and the International Monetary Fund (Fuller 2012). It is worth noting that the historical context of organisations such as the World Bank and the United Nations has led many communities, even to this day, to be sceptical of the motives of outside organisations even in the form of aid, development and global health initiatives.

Commentators such as Roy (2004), Said (1979), Freire (1996) and Fanon (2008) have discussed at length the intricacies of empire, colonisation and the 'other' on societies, people and places with discourses relating to the perception of East versus West and the apparent 'clash of civilisations' that renders values of the East flagrantly at odds with those of the West. Whilst Verma (2002), in reference to the Association of South East Asian countries (ASEAN), discusses the move towards intrinsic 'Asian values', drawing 'cultural boundaries between the West and Asian countries'.

Understanding colonialism as a historical context is commented on by a number of Malaysian academics who note how this period is crucial to understanding certain issues today, including those relating to sexuality, and that the legacies both of

© The Author(s) 2018
S. Barmania, M.J. Reiss, *Islam and Health Policies Related
to HIV Prevention in Malaysia*, SpringerBriefs in Public Health,
https://doi.org/10.1007/978-3-319-68909-8_2

being a former British colony and of being a Muslim majority state are highly significant (Shah 2012). In addition, academics, such as Lee, argue that Malaysia's
evolution towards technology, globalisation and capitalism has an important role
(Lee 2011). The predominant religion in the country is Islam, of the Ibn Shafi school
of thought, which has a ubiquitous influence on Malay society and everyday life. In
addition, as Malaysian academic Shah describes, Islam is also a 'powerful shaper of
policies and public opinion in Malaysia' (Shah 2012), which often relate to sexuality and HIV. Nevertheless, before delving into these areas further, we provide a
succinct update on the HIV epidemic globally, within the Muslim world and in the
Asia Pacific region.

The Global HIV Epidemic, the Muslim World and Asia Pacific

It is estimated that in 2016, there were 36.7 million people living with HIV globally
and 1.8 million people newly infected with HIV (UNAIDS 2017). The HIV epidemic is characterised by rapid geographical changes in its disease dynamics as
well as breaking new grounds in science, both in treatment and prevention.
Notwithstanding this, HIV has also been a disease that has been surrounded by fear,
controversy, stigma and discrimination; this has particularly been the case when
associations between morality and religion have occurred. HIV has affected many
communities associated with a religious affinity, including those who affiliate themselves with Islam and the Muslim world.

However, the epidemiological evidence does suggest that HIV prevalence is
lower amongst Muslims (Gray 2003). Limits on sexual activity may have an influence on transmission of sexually transmitted diseases; the following of certain
Islamic rulings, if adhered to, such as male circumcision, can reduce transmission
of HIV. In the analysis conducted by Gray of existing research with Muslim populations in Sub-Saharan Africa, which including 38 studies, six of seven studies
observed a negative relationship between HIV prevalence and Islam. A study in
Kenya showed that male circumcision, often a requirement of certain religious
groups, 'significantly reduces the risk of HIV acquisition in young men in Africa'
(Bailey et al. 2007). The protective effect was estimated to be in the region of 60%
and male circumcision has been rolled out in many parts of Africa. In addition, a
study by Kagimu et al. (2012) undertaken in Uganda showed that *sujda* (a mark on
the forehead caused by repeatedly prostrating in prayer) and fasting were associated
with lower HIV infections.

The Middle East is often considered the epicentre of the Muslim World and frequently anecdotally classed as a place where 'HIV does not exist'. Obermeyer discusses the low prevalence of HIV in the Middle East and also recognises that there
is 'no room for complacency' with some of the earlier views revealing a denial of the
existence of HIV in the region and the perception that HIV was imported from other
countries which were sexually immoral and that Islam itself was protection enough
(Obermeyer 2006). Furthermore, Obermeyer examined how some of the practices

that were routine amongst Muslims resulted in decreased HIV transmission; these practices included low alcohol intake, which reduces disinhibition and risky behaviour, as well as male circumcision, whilst other practices, such as moralizing, gender inequality and vulnerability of women, had rather more negative results.

Nevertheless, there is a growing realization that the Middle East and North Africa 'are not immune to HIV' and consequently there has been an engagement with religious leaders, imams, priests and civil society as well as those affected with HIV to train imams and priests to sensitize the congregation about HIV, including Friday sermons (El Feki 2006). However, there is a big gulf between those people who have acquired HIV through 'respectable' avenues such as blood transfusions than those who have acquired HIV through means that are deemed less palatable.

In 2010, Abu-Raddad and colleagues undertook a systematic review of studies relating to HIV, Sexually Transmitted Infections (STIs) and risk behaviours in the Middle East and North Africa and found that there was evidence of HIV prevalence in certain high risk groups such as IVDUs (Intravenous drug users), Men who had Sex with Men (MSM) and female sex workers (Abu-Raddad et al. 2010). The study also showed that MSM were the most hidden and stigmatized of all HIV groups in the Middle East and North Africa, with low levels of condom use; they served as a bridging population (a population that carries HIV in high incidence groups to the rest of society) and included fishermen, truck drivers and the clients of sex workers. More recently, Mumtaz and colleagues conducted a review of HIV in the Middle East and North African region which showed that there are new data to suggest that there are growing HIV epidemics in key populations such as MSM, IVDUs and female sex workers with a low prevalence elsewhere (Mumtaz et al. 2014). It has been estimated that within the region concentrated HIV epidemics are emerging amongst MSM, with up to 28% of those living with HIV being from the MSM community (Mumtaz et al. 2011). Yet, in many parts of the Middle East and North Africa there is legislation against Men who have Sex with Men making it difficult for health care workers to tackle HIV; whilst some countries such as Lebanon, Tunisia and Morocco have been more open to dealing with these issues, other countries can be more hostile (Burki 2011). Although the World Health Organisation has guidelines against discrimination against Men who have Sex with Men, these are not always implemented in many countries (WHO 2011).

Rajabali and colleagues discuss HIV and Men who have Sex with Men in Pakistan, another Muslim country where culture and society impact on everyday life, including that of sexual life, where sex outside marriage and homosexuality are taboo; thus, many believe that HIV 'cannot be a problem in the Muslim world' (Rajabali et al. 2008). The authors highlight the fact that although these practices are considered against Islam the condemnation serves to drive behaviour underground and places policy makers in a predicament of how best to respond (Rajabali et al. 2008). Furthermore, there were myths that anal sex does not constitute 'having sex' and that carrying a condom was difficult, with only 32% of MSM reporting using a condom at last sexual interaction (Rajabali et al. 2008).

Notwithstanding this, the Muslim World is not homogenous; society and cultural attitudes vary depending on the region, whether it is the Middle East and North

Africa or countries within the Indian subcontinent such as Pakistan. However, the factor of Islam, or at least the perception of Islam and how it should be practised, contributes to issues such as denial, moralization and some structural issues which influence HIV prevention to a greater or lesser degree. Furthermore, many of the issues highlighted are similar to those experienced in Malaysia and other countries in South East Asia, which will be discussed later in the course of this chapter.

UNAIDS estimates that in Asia and the Pacific in 2016 there were 5.1 million people living with HIV and 270,000 new HIV infections (UNAIDS 2017). In addition, UNAIDS describes the response to HIV/AIDS in Asia Pacific as 'mixed', with areas of definitive progress in terms of a reduction of new HIV infections, while there are also growing epidemics among key populations such as MSM, so that there is a need to target HIV prevention activities on the key populations at highest risk (UNAIDS 2013). Dokubo et al. (2013) conducted a systematic review which highlighted the high HIV incidence among commercial sex workers, intravenous drug users and Men who have Sex with Men. In addition, factors associated with HIV infection among MSM included having multiple sexual partners, receptive anal sex and syphilis infection either currently or historically, whereas in the general population the factors were engaging in sexual activities with commercial sex workers, not using condoms during sex consistently and multiple sexual partners as well as recent genital ulceration.

HIV in Malaysia and High Risk Groups

The first case of HIV in Malaysia was documented in 1987 (Goh et al. 1987) and by December 1990 there were 750 cases of HIV infection, predominantly amongst drug users. Brettle (1992) first described some of the problems associated with HIV infection in Malaysia in the early '90s, including a 'reluctance to discuss sexual and drug related matters which is partly based on the teachings of Islam' and warned that Malaysia had to find a solution which would be acceptable to an Islamic society; those issues are just as relevant now as they were then (Barmania and Aljunid 2016).

The HIV/AIDS epidemic in Malaysia is focused mainly on at risk populations comprising Intra Venous Drug Users (IVDUs), sex workers and the transgender population (UNGASS 2012). In the early days of the epidemic in Malaysia, IVDU was the main driver of the epidemic; however, now there is a shift towards sexual transmission and in 2011 sexual transmission became the main driver of HIV infection with ratio of six sexual transmissions for every four as a result of IVDU transmissions (UNGASS 2012), most likely the result of harm reduction programmes for IVDU and needle exchange. Although, IVDUs are still considered a high risk group in Malaysia, other high risk groups include transgender (TG) individuals, Men who have Sex with Men (MSM) and Sex Workers; increasingly, Malaysian women are considered vulnerable to HIV with the feminization of the epidemic (Talib 2006).

Malaysia is marked by confined epidemics amongst key populations, such as IVDUs, MSM, sex workers, transgender individuals and vulnerable women. With regards to intravenous drug users, Malaysia is considered a country that has a 'mega epidemic' of HIV (Beyrer et al. 2010). However, in high risk groups there may often be an overlap between one subpopulation and another or one group may have multiple high risks.

Men Who Have Sex with Men

A major series on HIV amongst MSM highlighted the need to focus on this key group (Beyrer et al. 2012). In addition, Beyrer and colleagues undertook another review which showed that there are epidemics of HIV in MSM communities amongst most low, middle and upper income countries, with current prevention strategies ill-equipped to deal with such a spread, complicated by factors such as high numbers of sexual partners and intoxicant use during sex (Beyrer et al. 2013). In addition, there are a number of biological factors that predispose MSM to being vulnerable: the high transmission efficiency of receptive anal intercourse, the fact that men unlike women can be both receptive of anal sex (high risk for acquiring HIV) and insertive for anal sex (high risk for transmission of HIV), plus the large MSM networks (Beyrer et al. 2013). There are also social and structural factors such as denial and stigma towards MSM and limited funding for such groups that make access to such HIV prevention services and there existence in the first place more difficult (Beyrer et al. 2013).

In Asia the prevalence of HIV amongst Men who have Sex with Men is rising (Lim and Chan 2011) with associations of additional risky practices such as illicit drug use (Wei et al. 2012). Furthermore, amongst MSM in Asian countries such as Malaysia, those who are MSM are often 'hidden' and less likely to disclose their sexual behaviour, more likely to favour opting for HIV testing in community-based centres rather than health care based settings, in part due to culture and stigma (Koh and Kamarulzaman 2011). Furthermore, in Malaysia, despite the incidence of HIV transmission as a result of male-to-male sex being 19%, only 0.2% of the total HIV prevention budget was devoted to this specific high risk group (UNAIDS 2013).

More recently, there have been a couple of bio behavioural surveillance studies looking at MSM in Malaysia. Kanter and colleagues undertook a studying looking at the risk behaviours and HIV prevalence among 517 Men who have Sex with Men in Kuala Lumpur recruited through venues which MSM are likely to frequent, such as clubs, massage parlours, saunas and a park; 47% of these individuals were Muslim (Kanter et al. 2011). 3.9% of those tested positive for HIV and some of the common risk behaviours included unprotected anal sex with a steady male partner, unprotected receptive anal sex with more than one partner and anal sex under the influence of alcohol or recreational drugs, referred to colloquially as 'chem sex' (Bourne et al. 2014). The study concluded that there was a 'clear and urgent need' to provide HIV education within the MSM community and that while groups such as the Pink Triangle Foundation have the relevant connections with the community they serve, they are limited with respect to financial and technical resources. In addition, Malays were more likely than their Chinese counterparts to be HIV positive and engage in unprotected anal sex with a casual male partner.

Another multi-ethnic study looked at the prevalence of unprotected sex among MSM in Penang; out of a convenience sample of 350, 284 were Malay, with the most common means of finding sexual partners being through the internet (Lim et al. 2013). Forty percent of participants had not been exposed to any form of prevention activities or information and 70% had never been tested for HIV, while most participants (over 80%) had unprotected anal intercourse. It was concluded that active surveillance amongst MSM is required; there was also speculation of the possibility of an 'explosive HIV epidemic among MSM' which called for greater provision of HIV prevention within this group.

Koh and Yong looked at the perception of HIV risk amongst MSM at a community-based voluntary counselling and testing centre in Kuala Lumpur, operated by the Pink Triangle Foundation, a longstanding NGO which works with at risk communities including MSM (Koh and Yong 2014). Out of 423 clients who received voluntary counselling and testing, 8.5% (36 clients) described themselves as high risk, while 24 when tested were found to be HIV positive (9.4%), with a positive correlation seen between risk perception and HIV infection amongst clients. Clients who rated themselves as high risk for being infected with HIV were not only significantly associated with engaging in higher risk behaviour but were 17 times more likely to be infected with HIV than those who rated themselves as low risk. This is an important finding because it shows that MSM were able to perceive their risk accurately and given limited resources it is plausible that prevention strategies could be targeted for those who see themselves as being high risk, with the aim of altering sexual practices.

Furthermore, within the high risk group classed as MSM there are added high risk behaviours such as having unprotected receptive anal intercourse with internal ejaculation (Lim et al. 2012). Lim and colleagues undertook an internet study looking at 10,413 men across Asia; of the 7311 who had receptive anal intercourse, 47.5% had internal ejaculation and this was associated with less than high school education and use of the internet to seek sex partners. Malaysia was included in this study and it was found that Malaysia had high rates of unprotected receptive anal intercourse with internal ejaculation (51.9%) compared to the overall prevalence of 47.5%. The authors also conclude that in more traditional groups, culture and religion can make MSM less likely to be involved in prevention programmes for fear of being found out as being gay, and so constitutes a lost opportunity.

In fact, the Asia Pacific Coalition on Male (APCOM) sexual health concluded that Islam influences both how homosexuality is viewed by the general public, sexual risk taking behaviours by MSM and also contributes to a fatalistic idea that HIV is their 'fate' MSM (APCOM 2012b discussion paper). Furthermore, Malay Muslim MSM, due to social and cultural pressures, may engage in intercourse with female partners for fear of looking out of place amongst their community (APCOM 2012a country brief). In addition, the coalition discusses Islam and sexual diversity and access to health services in their discussion paper and claims that Orthodox Islam has an overwhelmingly powerful influence on Muslims. They argue that the story of

Sodom and Gomorrah (story of Lot) is the cornerstone of the condemnation of homosexuality by the Abrahamic faiths; however, another reading is that the people of Lot were destroyed because of exploitation, xenophobia and sexual coercion of men (APCOM 2012b discussion paper). In any case, it is the conflicting identities of having sex with men and being a Muslim that can make MSM more vulnerable to HIV; by being forced into heterosexual marriage because of social pressure, they can seek extra-marital affairs as an outlet in the form of having sex with strangers, multiple partners or paid sex, thus being more vulnerable to HIV infection. Furthermore, associated guilt and self-stigmatisation can affect mental health, leading to depression, anxiety and suicide (APCOM 2012a; 2012b).

However, some authors argue that without a progressive opinion, the only two options for a same sex Muslim would be to convert to heterosexual behaviour or reject Islamic society. Some have concluded that same 'sex sexuality is put on the same level as adultery and/or fornication; it is not worse than either of these two activities' and is a 'sin like any other' (Jamal 2008). There are more progressive interpretations of the Story of Lot from both the Hebrew bible and the Qur'an. Nevertheless, such progressive interpretations are generally seen as an abomination to the majority of Muslims. All this highlights two main points: firstly, that there are differing perceptions of Islamic practice, along the progressive-conservative spectrum; and secondly that such condemnation may make MSM question their faith to such an extent that they chose to leave Islam altogether, a sin that is considered graver than any other.

Female Sex Workers

Another key group considered to be particularly vulnerable to HIV in Malaysia are sex workers (UNGASS 2014). A comprehensive systematic review and meta-analysis of the global burden of HIV among female sex workers in low and middle income countries was undertaken by Baral and colleagues which included Malaysia in its analysis (Baral et al. 2012). The study highlighted that although HIV infection in female sex workers varies across the region, there is a substantial increase in the odds ratio of HIV amongst sex workers compared to the general female population (Baral et al. 2012). Malaysia was found, based on the IBISS 2009 report, to have an odds ratio compared with HIV prevalence among the general female population of 81; HIV prevalence amongst sex workers in Malaysia was found to be 10.7% in a sample of 552 (IBISS 2009). The Baral et al. study concluded that there was an 'urgent need to scale up access to quality HIV prevention programming' as well as taking into consideration some of the structural and societal environments, stigma, discrimination and legalities that sex workers are faced with (Baral et al. 2013; Baral et al. 2014). There is a growing consensus that sex work is work, and that a greater emphasis should be placed on providing access to health care rather than moralising those in the industry (Empower 2012).

Transgender Women

Another of the key groups considered to be high risk of acquiring HIV in Malaysia are transgender women, those assigned male at birth but who identify with being women. Baral and colleagues recently undertook a meta-analysis and systematic review to assess the relative HIV burden in transgender women worldwide including in countries within the Asia Pacific region (Baral et al. 2012). The authors found the pooled HIV prevalence to be 19.1% in 11,066 women worldwide; in 7197 transgender women sampled in ten low and middle income countries the HIV prevalence was 17.7% and the odds ratio for being infected with HIV in transgender women compared with all adults of reproductive age across the 15 countries was 48.8. The authors also noted that transgender women were often not included in national HIV surveillance, yet prove a 'very high burden population for HIV', requiring 'urgent need of prevention'; transgender women often engage in high risk receptive anal sex with men, making them more vulnerable to acquiring HIV as well as being susceptible to stigma and discrimination in health care settings which acts to hinder access to prevention and treatment. In Malaysia, the local term for male to female transgender women is 'mak nyah' and it is estimated that there are 10,000–20,000 in the country, with the majority being Malay Muslims (Teh 2008). In 2002, Teh studied 507 mak nyah and found that over 92% received payment for sex, although only 54% claimed they were sex workers; the study was the first large scale piece of research to assess HIV/AIDS knowledge amongst this group (Teh 2002). Teh also undertook research in 2007 with 15 mak nyah in Malaysia and found that all respondents had heard of HIV/AIDS but lacked in-depth information and that this was not of paramount concern to them when compared to primary problems of employment and discrimination (Teh 2008). In addition, although condoms were carried they were seldom used due to issues such as clients' refusal, getting paid more for not using condoms, oral sex or perceptions of clients' health (Teh 2008). Overall, there has been a dearth of research regarding HIV amongst transgender women in Malaysia, although there has been some research regarding human rights.

Some have argued that historically transgender women were more accepted in Malaysian society than today (Lee 2011). Research conducted among members of the Lesbian, Gay, Bisexual and Transgender (LGBT) community in Malaysia including 13 transgender women found that they were subject to discrimination by Islamic religious officials with some transgender women feeling reluctant to access medical services due to being verbally abused, stared at or ill-treated by health professionals (KRYSS 2012). Human Rights Watch (2014) published a report that recounted alleged human rights abuses against transgender people in Malaysia; it catalogued some of the issues relating to health care: inappropriate touching or refusing to touch transgender women as patients as well as the fact that many transgender women felt discriminated at school and had lower levels of education. More specifically, Human Rights Watch recommendations to the Ministry of Health included training for health personnel on non-discrimination towards transgender people, establishing a national task force on HIV through sexual transmission and conducting off-site HIV testing for transgender people in 'safe spaces'. It is estimated that the prevalence of HIV among transgender women in Malaysia is 5.7% and it has been suggested that this could be underreported or underestimated (UNGASS 2014). Although most religious leaders would conclude that there is no such thing as a third gender other than that of *khunsa* (indeterminate sex), Islamic scholar Professor Hashim Kamali does discuss the need to look at issues surrounding transgenderism and justice in Malaysia through the prism of compassion, fairness and science (Kamali 2011).

Vulnerable Women and Other Groups

In Asia promoting the rights of women and girls, including female sex workers, women who use drugs and transgender women and girls in general, is important for preventing HIV (UN Women 2013). Low and Wong (2014) state that the primary risk factor faced by women in acquiring HIV is their 'inability to control when and whether to be sexually active', with gender disparities at its foundation as well as forced and unsafe sex. A Malaysia country brief, specifically focussing on HIV and key affected women and girls, highlighted some of the social and economic factors that render Malaysian woman and girls more vulnerable to HIV, due to gender dynamics, the more submissive role of woman in society and a lack of awareness of HIV and AIDS (UN Women Malaysia 2013). In addition, due to economic factors and limited education, some women may enter into sex work for economic reasons; with little sex education, women may be less able to negotiate safer sex in such situations, including condom use and saying no altogether (UN Women Malaysia 2013).

Knowledge and Perceptions of HIV in Malaysia and of Sex Education

There have been a number of studies undertaken in Malaysia looking at the knowledge of people with regards to HIV and at perceptions towards those living with HIV. Jahanfar et al. (2010) looked at the sexual behaviour, knowledge and attitudes of non-medical university students towards HIV/AIDS in Malaysia, undertaking a cross-sectional study amongst 530 university students randomly sampled using a self-administered questionnaire. Although knowledge was considered high amongst this group, information from parents and medical profession was found to be low and the main source was from the internet. Rahnama et al. (2011) undertook a cross-sectional study of 1773 respondents at a public university to assess attitudes surrounding HIV; only 19.5% said they would inform partners or family if diagnosed with HIV. Furthermore, the study found that 93% approved of screening for HIV as a prerequisite for marriage, feeling that it should be compulsory; 91.6% believed that premarital HIV testing can protect men and women from HIV.

Zulkifli and colleagues examined knowledge, attitudes and beliefs related to HIV among adolescents in Malaysia and found that although knowledge was high, there were misconceptions about HIV transmission (Zulkifli and Wong 2002). The authors concluded that knowing about HIV/AIDS is not protective in itself and call for a critical review of HIV prevention programmes which openly address risk taking behaviours without moral judgement. In addition, Wong, in a cross-sectional study of 2271 people in Malaysia, found that ethnicity was a factor in HIV transmission knowledge, with Malays scoring lower than other ethnicities (Wong 2013).

Various studies have looked at sex education in Malaysia. An analysis of sex education in schools across Malaysia was conducted in 2011; this sampled 380 university students and compared participants' own experience of sex education compared with the standard UNESCO technical guidelines on sexuality education which had been undertaken by the students (Talib et al. 2012; UNESCO 2009). The authors categorically stated that 'it can be said in its entirety that sex education is not taught in classes across the nation', based on their finding that 85% of respondents felt that current teaching was 'unclear' and 'limited', even though sexuality education was provided in schools often in Science, Biology or Islamic studies classes. Ninety percent of those respondents felt that sexuality education should be implemented in Malaysian schools, taught separately (as a subject) at form 3 and relating it to an Islamic perspective (Talib et al. 2012). Sex education was examined by Low and colleagues who undertook a qualitative study of 31 Malaysian adolescent boys between the ages of 13 and 17 years in Klang valley; they concluded that in Malaysia programmes referring to sexual health were 'scanty' (Low et al. 2007). Boys were found still to hold onto traditional views that sex should only be between husband and wife, sexual activity should be deferred till marriage and 'premarital sex only happened in the West'. Conforming to social norm, parents were categorically not a source of information; rather, peers, the internet and newspapers were cited instead.

Harm Reduction in Malaysia

Malaysia started to follow in the footsteps of other countries by proposing harm reduction in response to increasing cases of HIV with a Needle Syringe Programme (NSP) and Methadone Maintenance Therapy (MMT) (Rao 2010). These were seen to be against the teachings of Islam and some feared they would encourage drug use, but subsequently Malaysia has been looked upon favourably in terms of its political leadership, commitment and partnership, with Rao commending Malaysia for its supportive role in implementing needle exchange from 2005. In fact, other countries such as Bangladesh and Maldives have undertaken study visits to Malaysia with the aim of learning and replicating good practice in their own countries. They chart that coverage has even included mosques, noting that as a Muslim majority population 'the involvement of the religious organizations and leaders has played a pivotal role in gaining support for the harm reduction program in the country' (World Bank 2011). Furthermore, in 2013 the World Bank group undertook an extensive cost effectiveness analysis study of the harm reduction programme in Malaysia and concluded that the "MMT and NSP as implemented in Malaysia are cost effective and are expected to produce net cost savings to the government in the future" and continued as a strategy to limit the transmission of HIV among those people who inject drugs (World Bank 2014). However, as Reid and colleagues explain, the introduction of harm reduction and needle exchange programmes was not without its challenges, with the government initially rejecting the proposal, deeming it would encourage drug use; however, due to NGO pressure there was a shift in the government, although still difficulty promoting such a stance amongst Islamic religious leaders (Reid et al. 2007).

Kamarulzaman and colleagues discuss the issues of Islam and harm reduction, highlighting the tensions given that drug abuse is forbidden yet drug use is prevalent in many Muslim countries, as is HIV. They utilised Islamic principles such as the importance of preservation of man and limiting harm (*darar*), and in some situations 'a lesser harm may be tolerated to eliminate a greater harm' as well as the principle of '*maslaha*', that public interest should be prioritized over personal interests, to justify harm reduction (Kamarulzaman and Saifuddeen 2009). Important as many objections to HIV prevention approaches are, due to objections on Islamic grounds or anticipated objections, Islam has always been practical and forward thinking and there exists a complex set of principles which are available for promoting harm reduction in Muslim countries (Kamarulzaman and Saifuddeen 2009). Todd and colleagues argue for 'harm reduction adapted to the context of the local culture' and argue that although Islam is against premarital sex and intoxicant use, it is also not 'monolithic'; they argue for greater dialogue between harm reduction providers and religious leaders with an emphasis on Islamic beliefs in mercy (Todd et al. 2007).

Memoona Hasnain (2005) highlights some of the cultural issues such as the foreboding role of religious leaders and the gap between Islamic theory and practice. Hassnain also highlights that countries with a high HIV prevalence, such as Uganda, have concluded that the need to preserve life overrides the sin, if any, of using condoms. Narayan and colleagues explain how the current drug policy in Malaysia came about, slowly and with great difficulty; the NGOs were fundamental in producing change and is important to learn from history with a view to reducing the sexual transmission of HIV (Narayan et al. 2011). The authors critically examine the forces and factors that ultimately caused a transition from the punitive approach that had previously existed; ultimately, there was something of a competition between three stakeholders: the state, a vocal Muslim lobby and the NGOs. This took place within a growing acknowledgment that the attempts at the time to curb HIV were simply not effective enough. Notwithstanding this, although great strides have been made in harm reduction amongst IVDUs, utilising Islamic principles of preservation of life, the same cannot be said of prevention of HIV attributed to sexual transmission (Science 2014); this remains significantly underfunded in comparison (Kamarulzaman 2013).

Islamic Engagement

In general, there has been a lack of engagement by Muslims and Muslim organisations with HIV, one argument for why this is provided by Eekelen and Mould (2011):

> Few development organisations with a Muslim identity work in the field of HIV. This is largely because HIV is associated with drugs and sex outside marriage, and therefore has the potential of alienating the organisations' sponsors and employees.

A further barrier to effective engagement is that Muslim affiliated organisations and professionals can find it hard to integrate and access the highly secular 'HIV world', such as the International Aids Conference; yet, by not participating they essentially ostracise themselves as 'meaningful stakeholders'. However, Islamic jurisprudence has been utilized in HIV prevention, for example, *ikhtiar akhaffadararain* or choosing 'the lesser of two evils', as well as principles of mercy and forgiveness to counteract stigma and discrimination:

> Allah's Messenger (may peace be upon him) said: A prostitute saw a dog moving around a well on a hot day and hanging out its tongue because of thirst. She drew water for it in her shoe and she was pardoned (for this act of hers) (Hadith from Muslim. Book 26, Chapter 38, 5578)

> Whoever kills a human being … it shall be as though he had killed all mankind; and that whoever saves a human life, it shall be as though he had saved the life of all mankind. (Al Quran, Surah al Maidah, Chapter 5, Verse 32)

Religious professionals have the potential to use *khutbahs*, religious classes, pre-marital courses and religious radio programmes to disseminate information as they are respected and trusted in the community to deliver accurate information. Often, religious leaders are reluctant to speak about social issues such as HIV as they fear that 'speaking about the illicit reality of sex is tantamount to doing it' (Long 2009). Religious leaders have been key players in the fight against HIV in predominantly Muslim regions, such as the Middle East (McGirk 2008) and were identified as one of the key stakeholders and potential advocates in the fight against HIV/AIDS (Kanda et al. 2013; UNDP 2006).

There have been other ways in which an Islamic approach to tackling HIV has been proposed, such as incorporating the evidence of the *Qu'ran* and *Hadith* (Ibrahim 2014), even justifying condom usage under the ruling that 'necessity permits the forbidden', but ultimately an effective prevention strategy is believed to be following Islam itself, demonstrating a direct linkage between power, religion and policy. Many believe that Islamic religious leaders should be involved in HIV prevention. In 2011, the Malaysian AIDS Council produced a short report titled *Responsible religious response to HIV and AIDS in Malaysia* calling for a 'greater involvement by religious authorities' (MAC 2011). MAC partnered with religious departments at both national and state levels, including JAKIM (the religious policy making department). Subsequently, they produced the HIV and Islam programme in 2009, the objectives of which were to increase political leadership amongst Muslim leader efforts to educate religious leaders, to tackle stigma and discrimination and to harmonise efforts with other stakeholders. The HIV and Islam manual (JAKIM 2011) provided training for religious leaders on issues such as spreading AIDS awareness and preventing HIV from an Islamic perspective, and produced practical guidelines on funeral rituals and a reiteration of the message against stigma and discrimination (MAC 2011). In addition, it helped with training religious leaders and conducting workshops nationwide and ensuring a greater profile for HIV on World Aids Day in mosques and in Friday *khutbahs*. It is also worth noting that the role of Islamic leaders in Malaysia differs compared to some other Muslim countries as these leaders are governed and salaried by a central authority, introducing a new power dynamic.

Access to HIV Services and the Importance of Environment

Dangerfield et al. (2015) undertook a study looking at the awareness and utilization of the HIV services of an AIDS community-based organisation, the PT Foundation, in Kuala Lumpur from 614 MSM who were reached through their own outreach services. Amongst them nearly half had never heard of the PT Foundation, of those who had heard of the organization 12.9% had visited it and 63.2% of MSM on out-reach believed they didn't know about HIV transmission. The authors acknowledge that having an organisation such as the PT Foundation which is managed by the MSM community makes it more sensitive to their needs (Dangerfield et al. 2015). Providing HIV prevention to populations that are most at risk, such as IVDUs, MSM and sex workers, combined with stigma and criminalization can make access to services for these groups difficult (Beyrer et al. 2011). Furthermore, potential service users become reluctant to utilise existing services, rendering those at highest risk less able to access care (Beyrer et al. 2011). Certain atmospheres can facilitate or hinder access to HIV prevention services, as well as wider issues such as the social environment and the law. There has been interest by authors and social scientists such as Auerbach regarding the structural and social interventions available to prevent HIV, such as laws and institutions to create enabling environments where individuals can protect themselves from HIV (Auerbach 2009). However, there is an awareness that changing social norms, laws and policies takes time and often the social interventions that may be best placed to decrease the incidence of HIV are quite likely those that relate to marginalised groups such as sex workers where public support may be low. Thus, Auerbach cites the central dilemma that 'weighing public health imperatives against societal mores and norms involves uncomfortable political calculation that most elected officials would prefer to avoid'. There have also been calls for a rights-based approach to HIV programming and this looks at the legal and policy environment as well as the right to health, whether this is available and accessible and whether those who are vulnerable are reached (Gruskin and Tarantola 2008).

In Malaysia, a consultation was conducted in 2013 indicating that some of the current laws may not provide the ideal enabling environment for HIV services (UN

Malaysia 2014). Some of these laws pertained to Men who have Sex with Men ('*liwat*') and sex work (referred to in Malaysian law as prostitution), which are both offences against the national penal code and federal *Shariah* (in Malaysia termed Syariah) criminal system. In addition, under the Syariah criminal system any 'male posing as a woman for immoral purposes' is guilty of an offence (Syariah 1997); this is the Act mostly related to transgender women.

Condom Promotion and Premarital HIV Testing

In Malaysia it is commonly acknowledged that condom promotion is not significantly utilised as a means of HIV prevention (NCPI 2014); condom promotion is fragmented, sporadic, certainly not consistent. This approach by Malaysia with respect to condom usage differs substantially compared to the policy as stipulated by WHO, UNFPA and UNAIDS which cites condom use as a 'critical element' in HIV prevention and treatment and consider the latex condom to be the single most efficient method to reduce sexual transmission of HIV and advises it to be readily accessible (UNAIDS 2009). In fact, following a technical review the WHO concluded that there was a significant demand for additional lubricant, especially for MSM during anal intercourse to prevent condom breakage, whilst acknowledging that in the absence of such lubricants, products such as baby oil, lotions and petroleum jelly should not be used with condoms (WHO 2012).

One of the policies in place to prevent the spread of HIV in Malaysia is the premarital testing of prospective Muslim married couples. Johor was the first state in Malaysia to initiate screening in 2001. The rationale for the testing is as a means to limit the spread of HIV from spouse to spouse or to children. Tan and colleagues discuss the cost effectiveness of HIV screening in the general population in the form of premarital HIV testing and acknowledge there has not been any cost effective analysis on premarital HIV testing amongst Muslim couples (Tan and Koh 2008). However, the authors argue that the test is only useful at one point in time and does not guarantee that individuals may not be exposed in the future. Also, there are issues as to whether confidentiality can be kept when religious officers are involved and a marriage is not just the union of two individuals, but of two families.

Islamic scholar Professor Hashim Kamali in the early days of the implementation of the pre-marital HIV screening programme discussed the issues relating to mandatory HIV testing and the passing of the Johor Islamic Religious Council fatwa that made HIV testing compulsory for all Muslim couples planning to wed in Johor (Kamali 2001). He specified the justification as under the rule of '*maslaha*' (public interest), intended to protect 'religion, life, property, intellect and lineage'.

However, there have been objections on the grounds of human rights and by international organisations such as the WHO. Mandatory testing of HIV (as in the case of premarital HIV testing for Muslim married couples) is 'never sanctioned and is opposed by WHO, UNAIDS and UNHCR' (UNHCR 2014), although it notes that mandatory testing of blood, blood products or organs is ethical and necessary.

It has been argued that all HIV testing services should follow the '5 Cs' of informed consent, confidentiality, counselling, correct test results and connection to HIV services both those of prevention and those of treatment (UNHCR 2014). The Open Society Institute (Open Society 2000) has discussed the rising number of groups, including religious organisations and Muslim countries such as Bahrain and Saudi Arabia, that have adopted mandatory HIV premarital testing but maintains that such actions not only compromise the principles of HIV testing but are also against human rights, especially the right to marry and family.

In addition, some have argued against such policies in Asia and the Middle East, for example in India, arguing that there is the potential for increased risk of stigma and discrimination of those with HIV, of limiting women's rights as well as denigration of human rights, and have concluded that the ultimate responsibility lies with the individual (Malhotra et al. 2008). Malhotra and colleagues have also argued that the state's role is to create an enabling environment to obtain information about HIV and is 'conducive to voluntary counselling and testing, rather than through coercive mandatory testing strategies'.

Ganczak undertook a study showing the impact of premarital HIV testing from selected countries in the Arab peninsula and found that there was high social acceptability of HIV testing amongst young Emirates who showed a vulnerability to HIV (Ganczak 2010). Although in such Muslim countries premarital sex is contrary to the teachings of Islam, the acceptance of such a test acknowledges that some Muslims do engage in such activities and that testing may be an entry point and serve to provide a platform to educate on HIV/health issues and an opportunity for HIV surveillance.

Gruskin argues that for a rights-based approach to HIV there should be participation, which is free, active and includes the key affected communities and greater involvement of people living with HIV at 'every stage of HIV policy making and programming' and that this is seen as crucial for an effective response; however, this is often absent in many countries (Gruskin and Tarantola 2008). A strong civil society is important in creating changes in health policy, including in the HIV arena where civil organisations such as Treatment Action Campaign (Barmania and Lister 2013) have been vital. In addition, UNAIDS has guidelines on the participation of civil society to hold governments to 'account' and inclusion of PLHIV in policy making (UNAIDS 2011). This participation should extend to research and publication, says Choy (2014), who calls for the NGO community and advocacy groups in Malaysia to describe their work and successes to ensure leveraging of funds.

Conclusion

There has been growing appreciation that a 'one size fits all' model will not cater to all cultures and religious contexts and that religion itself can be utilised to help prevent disease (Husseini and Laporte 2001). While there has been a significant amount of research on HIV in Malaysia over the past 15 years (Choy 2014), there is little relating to the intersection of HIV and Islam in Malaysia. Religion, in this case Islam, needs to be taken seriously when thinking of how we deal with HIV in general and in a predominantly Muslim country in particular, such as Malaysia. The reasons for doing so are numerous and far reaching not just because there are links between Islam and behaviour but also because Islam affects the political and social environment. Some countries are able to navigate some of the more sensitive areas where Islam and public health intersect (Webster 2013); others may have more difficulty. Fundamentally, there are conflicting views on sexuality between the sexually liberal HIV community and the more conservative Muslim community, which can make it difficult for the latter to participate and engage with the former.

Notwithstanding this, there are some professionals from a Muslim background who have managed to navigate both worlds, i.e. the HIV community and the religious community, such as the Alaei brothers from Iran (McGirk 2008). This adds weight to the argument that such research/work needs to come from the inside, from those who understand the culture and context in order for policy change to be accepted by the local community; measures should be instigated from within the community rather than outside of it.

Islam and HIV prevention do not necessarily have to be at diametrically irreconcilable poles; there can, in fact, be a medium in between where collaboration and effective engagement are possible. Effective engagement in HIV research by Muslims for Muslims, where currently there is a paucity of knowledge, will ultimately improve practice and aid HIV prevention. This study adds to what is known about HIV in Muslim populations and specifically enters uncharted territory to look at the significance of religion to sexual health. This study critically analyses how Islam plays a role in shaping health policies and perceptions related to HIV prevention in Malaysia in the real world, charts how this role influences policy, process and power and examines how this influence is exerted both directly and indirectly in practice. The study takes a neutral perceptive, but addresses the gap of knowledge of Islam and HIV, examining how religion can be a determining factor to health— something which has hitherto been not extensively discussed.

References

Abu-Raddad, L., Hilmi, N., Mumtaz, G., Benkirane, M., Akala, F. A., Riedner, G., et al. (2010). Epidemiology of HIV infection in the Middle East and North Africa. *AIDS, 24*(Suppl 2), S5–S23.

APCOM. (2012a). *Country snapshots. Malaysia–HIV and men who have sex with men*. Bangkok: APCOM.

APCOM. (2012b). *Discussion paper: Islam, sexual diversity and access to health services*. Bangkok: APCOM.

Auerbach, J. (2009). Transforming social structures and environments to help HIV prevention. *Health Affairs, 28*(6), 1655–1665.

Bailey, R., Moses, S., Parker, C. B., Agot, K., Maclean, I., Krieger, J. N., et al. (2007). Male circumcision for HIV prevention in young men in Kisumu, Kenya: a randomised controlled trial. *Lancet, 369*(9562), 643–656.

Baral, S., Beyrer, C., Muessig, K., Poteat, T., Wirtz, A. L., Decker, M. R., et al. (2012). Burden of HIV among female sex workers in low income and middle income countries: a systematic review and meta-analysis. *Lancet Infectious Diseases, 12*, 538–549.

Baral, S., Claire, E., Shannon, K., Logie, C., Semugoma, P., Sithole, B., et al. (2014). Enhancing benefits or increasing harms: community responses for HIV among men who have sex with men, transgender women, female sex workers, and people who inject drugs. *Journal of Acquired Immune Deficiency Syndrome, 66*(Suppl 3), S319–S328.

Baral, S., Poteat, T., Stromdahl, S., Wirtz, A. L., Guadamuz, T. E., & Beyrer, C. (2013). Worldwide burden of HIV in transgender women: as systematic review and meta-analysis. *Lancet Infectious Diseases, 13*, 214–222.

Barmania, S., & Aljunid, S. M. (2016). Navigating HIV prevention policy and Islam in Malaysia: contention, compatibility or reconciliation? Findings from in-depth interviews among key stakeholders. *BMC Public Health, 16*, 524.

Barmania, S., & Lister, G. (2013). Civil society organisations, global health governance and public diplomacy. In I. I. Kichbusch (Ed.), *Global health diplomacy: Concepts, issues, actors, instruments, fora and cases* (pp. 253–267). New York: Springer.

Beyrer, C., Baral, S., Kerrigan, D., El-Bassel, N., Bekker, L. G., & Celentano, D. D. (2011). Expanding the space: Inclusion of most at risk populations in HIV prevention, treatment and care services. *Journal of Acquired Immune Deficiency Syndrome, 57*(Suppl 2), S96–S99.

Beyrer, C., Baral, S., Van Griensven, F., Goodreau, S. M., Chariyalertsak, S., Wirtz, A. L., et al. (2012). Global epidemiology of HIV infection in men who have sex with men. *Lancet, 380*(9839), 367–377.

Beyrer, C., Sullivan, P., Sanchez, J., Baral, S., Collins, C., Wirtz, A., et al. (2013). The global HIV epidemics in men who have sex with men (MSM): Time to act. *AIDS, 27*, 2665–2678.

Beyrer, C., Malinowska-Sempruch, K., Kamarulzaman, A., Kazatchkine, M., Sidibe, M., & Strathdee, S. A. (2010). HIV in people who use drugs-a time to act: A call for comprehensive responses to HIV in people who use drugs. *Lancet, 376*, 552–563.

Bourne, A., Reid, D., Hickson, F., Torres Rueda, S., & Weatherburn, P. (2014). *The chemsex study: Drug use in sexual settings among gay and bisexual men in Lambeth, Southwark and Lewisham*. London: Sigma Research (London School of Hygiene and Tropical Medicine).

Brettle, R. P. (1992). Observations of the problems of HIV infection in Malaysia. *Journal of Infection, 24*, 101–102.

Burki, T. (2011). HIV in men who have sex with men in the Middle East. *Lancet Infectious Diseases, 11*, 734–735.

Choy, K. K. (2014). A review of HIV/AIDS research in Malaysia. *Medical Journal of Malaysia, 69*(Supple A), 68–81.

Dangerfield, D., Gravitt, P., Rompalo, A., Yap, I., Tai, R., & Lim, S. H. (2015). Awareness and utilization of HIV services of an AIDS community based organisation in Kuala Lumpur, Malaysia. *International Journal or STD and AIDS, 26*(1), 20–26.

Dokubo, E. K., Kim, A. A., Le, L., Nadol, P. J., Prybylski, D., & Wolfe, M. I. (2013). HIV incidence in Asia: A review of available data and assessment of the epidemic. *AIDS Review, 15*, 67–76.

Eekelen, V., & Mould, H. (2011). In G. Ter Haar (Ed.), *Religion and development: Ways of transforming the world*. London: Hurst and Company.

El Feki, S. (2006). Middle Eastern AIDS efforts are starting to tackle taboos. *The Lancet, 367*, 975–976.

Empower. (2012). *Hit and run- sex worker's research on anti-trafficking in Thailand by Empower foundation*. Nontaburi: Empower University Press.

Fanon, F. (2008). *Black skin, white masks*. New York: Grove Press.

Freire, P. (1996). *Pedagogy of the oppressed*. London: Penguin Books.

Fuller, G. E. (2012). *A World without Islam*. New York: Back Bay Books.

Ganczak, M. (2010). The impact of premarital HIV testing: A perspective from selected countries from the Arabian Peninsula. *AIDS Care, 22*(11), 1428–1433.

Goh, K. L., Chua, C. T., Chiew, I. S., & Soo-Hoo, T. S. (1987). Acquired immune deficiency syndrome: A report of the first case in Malaysia. *Medical Journal of Malaysia, 42*(1), 58–60.

Gray, P. (2003). HIV and Islam: Is HIV prevalence lower among Muslims? *Social Science and Medicine, 58*(9), 1751–1756.

Gruskin, S., & Tarantola, D. (2008). Universal access to HIV prevention, treatment and care: assessing the inclusion of human rights in international and national strategic plans. *AIDS, 22*, S123–S132.

Hadith. Hadith from Muslim, Book 26, Chapter 38, 5578. http://sunnah.com/

Hasnain, M. (2005). Cultural approaches to HIV/AIDS harm reduction in Muslim countries. *Harm Reduction Journal, 2*, 23.

Human Rights Watch. (2014). *'I'm scared to be a woman'- Human rights abuses against transgender people in Malaysia*. New York: Human Rights Watch.

Husseini, A., & LaPorte, R. E. (2001). Islam with the internet could do much to prevent disease. *British Medical Journal, 323*, 694.

IBISS. (2009). *Malaysia integrated bio-behavioural (IBISS) survey*. Kuala Lumpur: Malaysian AIDS Council.

Ibrahim, F. (2014). The Islamic approach in mitigating HIV/AIDS. *International Journal of Public Health and Clinical Sciences, 1*(2), 14–18.

Jahanfar, S., Sann, L. M., & Rampal, L. (2010). Sexual behaviour, knowledge and attitudes of non-medical university students towards HIV/AIDS in Malaysia. *Shiraz E Medical Journal, 11*(3), 122–136.

JAKIM. (2011). *Manual on HIV/AIDS in Islam (English version)*. Putrajaya: Department of Islamic Development Malaysia.

Jamal, A. (2008). The story of lot and the Qur'an's perception of the morality of same sex sexuality. *Journal of Homosexuality, 41*, 1–88.

Kagimu, M., Guwatudde, D., Rwabukwali, C., Kaye, S., Walakira, K., & Ainomugisha, D. (2012). Religiosity for HIV prevention in Uganda: a case study among Muslim youth in Wakiso district. *African Health Science, 12*(3), 282–290.

Kamali, H. (2001). The Johor fatwa on mandatory HIV testing. *IIUM Law Journal, 9*(2), 99–116.

Kamali, H. (2011, August 11). Transgenders and justice in Islam. *New Straits Times*.

Kamarulzaman, A. (2013). Fighting the HIV epidemic in the Islamic world. *Lancet, 381*, 2060.

Kamarulzaman, A., & Saifuddeen, S. M. (2009). Islam and harm reduction. *International Journal of Drug Policy, 21*(2), 115–118.

Kanda, K., Jayasinghe, A., Silva Tudor, K., Priyadarshani, N. G. W., Delpitiya, N. Y., Obayashi, Y., Arai, A., Gamage, C., & Tamashiro, H. (2013). Religious leaders as potential advocates for HIV/AIDS prevention among the general population in Sri Lanka. *Global Public Health, 8*(2), 159–173.

Kanter, J., Koh, C., Razali, K., Tai, R., Izenberg, J., Rajan, L., et al. (2011). Risk behaviour and HIV prevalence among men who have sex with men in a multi-ethnic society: a venue-based study in Kuala Lumpur, Malaysia. *International Journal of STD and AIDS, 22*, 30–37.

Koh, K. C., & Kamarulzaman, A. (2011). Profiles of men who have sex with men seeking anonymous voluntary HIV counselling and testing at a community based centre in Malaysia. *Medical Journal of Malaysia, 66*(5), 491–494.

Koh, K. K., & Yong, L. S. (2014). HIV risk perception, sexual behaviour, and HIV prevalence among men who have sex with men at a community based voluntary counselling and testing center in Kuala Lumpur, Malaysia. *Interdisciplinary Perspectives on Infectious diseases, 2014*, 1–6.

KRYSS. (2012). *Violence: Through the lens of lesbians, bisexual women and transgender people in Asia. Malaysia: On the record*. New York: Outright Action International. https://www.outrightinternational.org/content/violence-through-lens-lbt-people-asia

Lee, J. C. H. (2011). *Policing sexuality: Sex, society and the state*. London: Zed Books.

Lim, S. H., Bazazi, R., Sim, C., Choo, M., Altice, F. L., & Kamarulzaman, A. (2013). High rates of unprotected anal intercourse with regular and casual partners and associated risk factors in a sample of ethnic Malay men who have sex with men (MSM) in Penang, Malaysia. *Sexually Transmitted Infection, 89,* 642–649.

Lim, S. H., & Chan, R. (2011). HIV infection among men who have sex with men in East and South East Asia-Time for action. *Sexual Health, 8,* 5–8.

Lim, S. H., Guadamuz, T. E., Wei, C., Chan, R., & Koe, S. (2012). Factors associated with unprotected receptive anal intercourse with internal ejaculation among men who have sex with men in a large internet sample from Asia. *AIDS Behaviour, 16,* 1979–1987.

Long, K. H. (2009). On sex, sin, and silence: An Islamic theology of storytelling for AIDS awareness. In F. Esack & S. Chiddy (Eds.), *Islam and AIDS: Between scorn, pity and justice* (pp. 154–168). Oxford: One World.

Low, W. Y., Ng, C. J., Fadzil, K. S., & Ang, E. S. (2007). Sexual issues: Let's hear it from the Malaysian boys. *Journal of Men's Health and Gender, 4*(3), 283–291.

Low, W. Y., & Wong, Y. L. (2014). Sexual and reproductive health and rights, HIV/AIDS and public health. *Asia Pacific Journal of Public Health, 26*(2), 116–117.

Malaysian Aids Council (MAC). (2011). *HIV and Islam: Responsible religious response to HIV and AIDS in Malaysia.* Kuala Lumpur: Malaysian Aids Council.

Malhotra, R., Malhotra, C., & Sharma, N. (2008). Should there be mandatory testing for HIV prior to marriage in India? *Indian Journal of Medical Ethics, 5*(2), 70–74.

McGirk, J. (2008). Religious leaders fight against HIV in Middle East. *Lancet, 372*(9635), 279–280.

Mumtaz, G., Hilmi, N., McFarland, W., Kaplan, R. L., Akala, F. A., Semini, I., et al. (2011). Are HIV epidemics among men who have sex with men emerging in the Middle East and North Africa?: A systematic review and data synthesis. *PLOS Medicine, 8*(8), 23–45.

Mumtaz, G. R., Riedner, G., & Abu-Raddad, L. (2014). The emerging face of the HIV epidemic in the Middle East and North Africa. *Current Opinion in HIV and AIDS, 9,* 183–191.

Narayan, S., Vicknasingam, B., & Robson, N. (2011). Transitioning to harm reduction: Understanding the role of non-governmental organisation in Malaysia. *International Journal of Drug Policy, 22,* 311–317.

NCPI Malaysia. (2014). Malaysia report. National commitments and policies instrument. http://files.unaids.org/en/dataanalysis/knowyourresponse/ncpi/2014countries/Malaysia%20NCPI%202013.pdf

Obermeyer, C. (2006). HIV in the Middle East. Prevalence of HIV in the Middle East is low but there is no room for complacency. *British Medical Journal, 333,* 851–854.

Open Society Institute. (2000). *Mandatory premarital HIV testing: An overview.* New York: Open Society Foundations.

Qur'an- The noble Qur'an. https://quran.com/

Rahnama, R., Rampal, L., Lye, M., & Rahman, H. (2011). Factors influencing students attitudes towards HIV/AIDS in a public university, Malaysia. *Global Journal of Health Sciences, 3*(1), 128–134.

Rajabali, A., Khan, S., Warraich, H. J., Khanani, M. R., & Ali, S. H. (2008). HIV and homosexuality in Pakistan. *Lancet Infectious Disease, 8,* 511–515.

Rao, P. (2010). AIDS in Asia amid competing priorities: a review of national responses to HIV. *AIDS, 24*(Suppl 3), S41–S48.

Reid, G., Kamarulzaman, A., & Kaur, S. S. (2007). Malaysia and harm reduction: The challenges and responses. *International Journal of Drug Policy, 18,* 136–140.

Roy, A. (2004). *The ordinary person's guide to Empire.* London: Flamingo Books.

Said, E. (1979). *Orientalism.* London: Penguin Books.

Science. (2014). Malaysia tries to follow Australia's path. *Science, 345,* 6193.

Shah, S. (2012). The Malaysian dilemma: negotiating sexual diversity in a Muslim-majority commonwealth state. In C. Lennox & M. Waites (Eds.), *Human rights, sexual orientation and gender identity in the common wealth* (pp. 261–285). London: SAS Publications.

Syariah. (1997). *Laws of Malaysia Syariah criminal offences.* Federal Territories Act.

Talib, J., Mamat, M., Ibrahim, M., & Mohamad, Z. (2012). Analysis of sex education in schools across Malaysia. *Procedia – Social and Behavioral Sciences, 59,* 340–348.

Talib, R. (2006). *Malaysia: Fighting a rising tide: The response to AIDS in East Asia*. Tokyo: Japan Centre for International Exchange.

Tan, H. L., & Koh, L. C. (2008). Is HIV screening in the general population cost effective? *Malaysian Family Physician, 3*(2), 96–97.

Teh, Y. K. (2002). *The Mak Nyahs: Malaysian male to female transsexuals*. Singapore: Eastern University Press.

Teh, Y. K. (2008). HIV related needs for safety among male to female transsexuals (mak nyah) in Malaysia. *SAHARA-J Journal of Social Aspects of HIV/AIDS, 5*(4), 178–185.

Todd, C., Nassiramanesh, B., Stanekzai, M. R., & Kamarulzaman, A. (2007). Emerging HIV epidemics in Muslim countries: Assessment of different cultural responses to harm reduction and implications of HIV control. *Current HIV/AIDS Reports, 4*(4), 151–157.

UN Women. (2013). *Country briefs on HIV and key affected women and girls in ASEAN*. Bangkok: UN Women.

UN Women Malaysia. (2013). *Malaysia country brief – HIV and key affected women and girls*. Bangkok: UN Women.

UNAIDS. (2009). *Policy statement on condoms and HIV prevention*. Geneva: UNAIDS.

UNAIDS. (2011). *UNAIDS guidance for partnerships with civil society, including people living with HIV and key populations*. Geneva: UNAIDS.

UNAIDS. (2013). *HIV in Asia and the Pacific. UNAIDS report 2013*. Bangkok: UNAIDS.

UNAIDS. (2017). *Global HIV statistics*. Geneva: UNAIDS.

UNDP. (2006). *Role of religious leaders in the fight against HIV/AIDS*. New York: UNDP.

UNESCO. (2009). *International technical guidance on sexuality education: Volume 1 The rationale for sexuality education*. Paris: UNESCO.

UNGASS Malaysia. (2012). *Global AIDS response progress – Malaysia*. Putrajaya: Ministry of Health.

UNGASS Malaysia. (2014). *Global AIDS response progress –Malaysia*. Putrajaya: Ministry of Health.

UNHCR. (2014). *Policy statement on HIV testing and counselling for refugees and other persons of concern to UNHCR*. Geneva: UNHCR.

United Nations Malaysia. (2014). *The policy and legal environment related to HIV services in Malaysia: Review and consultation*. Kuala Lumpur: United Nations.

Verma, V. (2002). Debating rights in Malaysia: Contradictions and challenges. *Journal of Contemporary Asia, 32*(1), 108–130.

Webster. (2013). Indonesia: Islam and health. *Canadian Medical Association Journal, 185*, 2.

Wei, C., Guadamuz, T. E., Lim, S. H., Huang, Y., & Koe, S. (2012). Patterns and levels of illicit drug use among men who have sex with men in Asia. *Drug and Alcohol Dependence, 120*(1-3), 246–249.

WHO. (2011). *Guidelines on the prevention and treatment of STI among men who have sex with men*. Geneva: WHO.

WHO. (2012). *Use and procurement of additional lubricants for male and female condoms*. Geneva: WHO.

Wong, L. P. (2013). Prevalence and factors associated with HIV/AIDS related stigma and discriminatory attitudes: A cross sectional study. *Preventative Medicine, 57*, S60–S63.

World Bank. (2011). *The harm reduction study visit. Kuala Lumpur Malaysia. Evaluation report*. Scope Group: Kuala Lumpur.

World Bank. (2014). *Return on Investment and Cost-Effectiveness of Harm Reduction Program in Malaysia*. Washington: World Bank Group.

Zulkifli, S., & Wong, L. Y. (2002). Knowledge, attitudes and beliefs related to HIV/AIDS among adolescents in Malaysia. *Medical Journal of Malaysia, 57*, 1–23.

Chapter 3
Methodology

Qualitative Methodology

The main methodology was qualitative in nature, best suited to explore the experiences, attitudes and practices of people within their social context (Ling 2006; Pope et al. 2000). A diverse range of stakeholders were interviewed to avoid bias and to gather a greater understanding of the complex nature of the issues at hand. The study itself was limited to sexual behaviours relating to HIV prevention.

Location, Time, Participants, Sampling

The study focussed on Peninsular Malaysia, urban areas within the Klang valley region, which included Kuala Lumpur and Putrajaya. Participants comprised the three main stakeholder groups identified as being involved in HIV prevention policy in Malaysia: People Living with HIV; religious leaders; and officials from the Ministry of Health. The data were collected over a six month period, from June to December 2013, with interviews taking place from October after successful and documented ethical approval from National University of Malaysia research and ethics committee.

People living with HIV (PLHIV) included Men who have Sex with Men (MSM), transgender women, sex workers and women who have acquired HIV through heterosexual transmission, all of whom were Muslim. These participants were recruited through the network and assistance of the PT Foundation, a longstanding local Malaysian NGO based in Kuala Lumpur, which was aware of the full inclusion and exclusion criteria. The religious leader group included individuals from the *Sharia* Department, Mufti's office, Islamic academic institutions, and the Department of

© The Author(s) 2018
S. Barmania, M.J. Reiss, *Islam and Health Policies Related to HIV Prevention in Malaysia*, SpringerBriefs in Public Health, https://doi.org/10.1007/978-3-319-68909-8_3

Islamic Development (Jabatan Kemajuan Islam Malaysia, JAKIM) at national and state level.

The participants were recruited using purposive sampling techniques. Thirty five participants were interviewed and recruitment curtailed once theoretical saturation was reached, consistent with standard qualitative research methods (Glaser and Strauss 1967; Bloor and Wood 2006). Nineteen PLHIV were interviewed, which reflected the heterogeneity of the group. Eleven religious leaders were interviewed, covering the spectrum of progressive thought to more conservative Islamic view-points. Finally, five participants were interviewed from the Ministry of Health, which included those from national and state level at the uppermost level of power and influence. In this group, theoretical saturation was reached early on as there was a strong consensus of opinion amongst those from within the department as well as homogeneity of viewpoints.

The study had a number of inclusion criteria for participants to be eligible to participate in the study, both general specific to stakeholder group. Criteria included that participants were aged over 18 and resided within the Klang Valley region of Malaysia and that PLHIV were living with HIV for 1 year or more. Participants were excluded if they did not provide informed written consent.

Interviews were conducted in person (face to face) by the same researcher (SB); being semi-structured in nature, they allowed similar data to be collected, ensuring standardisation, as well as being responsive to interviewees' understanding and par-ticular circumstances. After a literature review, brainstorming and discussions with colleagues, a topic guide with key questions and prompts was created, refined and used during interviews. The topic guide included an introduction, key questions as well as those that probed, with both a start and end point. The introduction included assurance of confidentiality, set ground rules for the interview and provided an opportunity to ask questions. Opening questions included exploring participants' views on HIV, health in general and the importance of Islam. Further questions centred on participants' knowledge of HIV prevention and policies in Malaysia, as well as perceptions of sex outside marriage, Men who have Sex with Men and con-dom usage.

Consent of the interviewees was obtained both orally and via a written consent form with brief details of the study provided in both English and Bahasa Malaysia. For the most part, interviews were conducted in English; however, in some instances during the interview translation was sought from colleagues. Most interviews lasted around 60 min, but ranged in length. Great attention was made to ensure that the inter-viewer was dressed in religiously appropriate attire when attending meetings with religious leaders, which included covering of head and limbs to respect local customs. Utilisation of open-ended questions, prompts and probes were used as appropriate as well as ensuring that a good rapport was established during the interview and being cognizant of any potential sensitivity and unease, probing accordingly.

Each interview was digitally audio-recorded, with file downloaded and stored securely as well as listened to again to ensure the recording was vocally clear. Manual notes were made during the interview to document any significant non-verbal communication. In addition, notes were made after the interview in free form to express any issues that arose from the interview. The audio files were transcribed professionally by someone experienced with qualitative research interviews and public health matters and accustomed to sensitive information and issues of confidentiality. The transcriber was satisfied with the clarity of the digital recordings they received and Malay accents.

The analysis of the data was undertaken in a detailed and systematic way as soon as the data were collected and the recording of the interview listened to again to understand and familiarize the researcher with the data, often with additional notes being taken. After the transcriber had produced a copy of the interview in verbatim form, the Word document was checked and compared with the audio file to ensure the transcription was accurate. Each transcript was printed and re-read in detail on a line-by-line basis and then re-read, this time with annotations and emerging themes noted. After about a third of the full sample of 35 had been read, which comprised all three stakeholders, a framework analysis was crafted. This framework was used to read and analyse through all the interview transcripts from scratch and provided a method of categorizing the data into themes. In some instances, more thanone1 theme could be assigned to a particular quote, which was noted on the transcript and the most applicable theme was chosen.

These ten themes comprised: Islam's view of life, health and wellbeing; sex outside marriage; knowledge about HIV in general; current HIV prevention practices in Malaysia; condoms; transgender women; Men who have Sex with Men; law and authority; stakeholder relationships; and action to be taken. In addition, there were some overriding themes such as language.

Quantitative Methodology

Quantitative data were collected to complement the qualitative data, which had been obtained prior to commencement of the survey distribution.

Study Tools, Location and Time, Respondents

The quantitative aspect of the study focussed on the same geographical area as the qualitative component but was undertaken at a different time, over a four month period, from December 2013 to April 2014. Questionnaires were used, which produced a standard set of data for each subject which was then later analysed statistically. After identifying the three stakeholder groups involved in having a role in HIV prevention, participants from those target groups were asked to share their views, opinions and knowledge. Those individuals who completed the questionnaire were not the same individuals as those who were interviewed for the qualitative component of the study.

The target groups comprised of those from the three key stakeholders identified as having a role in HIV prevention policies in Malaysia, namely people living with HIV (PLHIV), religious leaders and staff from the Ministry of Health. People Living with HIV included Men who have Sex with Men (MSM), transgender women, sex workers and women who acquired HIV through heterosexual transmission. These participants were purposively recruited through the PT Foundation, based in Kuala Lumpur. Respondents from the Islamic religious leader group included Muftis, academics working in Islamic academic institutions as well as those from JAKIM. Officials from the Ministry of Health were also surveyed.

The eventual sample size (n = 252) is consistent with other similar published research from within the field that have used similar HIV surveys (e.g. Nije-Carr 2009). Purposive sampling techniques were employed to recruit participants from the three identified stakeholder groups. Purposive sampling techniques have been used in other similar studies within the HIV arena (e.g. Zou et al. 2009). Initially, a self-administered questionnaire, which was written in English and Malay, was distributed to a convenience sample of eligible volunteers to probe knowledge related to HIV. Following ethics approval, prior to data collection the researcher organized to meet with a 'key contact person' from each stakeholder/target group to explain the purpose of the study of this research and seek their approval; later, these same people were contacted as entry points to aid in the distribution and collection of the questionnaire. From within the PLHIV group, this was someone from the executive director of the PT Foundation; similar meetings were undertaken with a representative from the Ministry of Health and a representative of Islamic religious leaders.

Following these in-person or telephone discussions, on various dates the researcher physically handed the questionnaire to participants in person, whilst assuring them of full anonymity and confidentiality or handed multiples copies to the key contact person. The participants then returned the questionnaire, folded, to the 'key person' within a specific time frame or to the researcher directly. This approach was felt more likely to improve the response rate rather than using a postal questionnaire. In addition, each participant received a token thank you (chocolates) as a small show of appreciation for their time.

The criteria for those who were eligible to complete the questionnaire comprised both general requirements and those specific to the three sampled groups. General criteria stipulated that participants were over the age of 18, provided informed consent, were either English or Malay speaking and resided in the Klang Valley region of Malaysia. Criteria specific to religious leaders were that participants were Islamic religious leaders (which could include both women and men).

Individuals were excluded from the questionnaire if they were under the age of 18 or did not provide informed consent; under the PLHIV group, individuals were excluded if they most likely acquired HIV though intravenous drug use.

An abridged bilingual version of the HIV Knowledge questionnaire developed by Wong et al. (2008), used previously in a Malaysian context, was validated and used with the permission of the authors. The questionnaire included basic demographic questions, including gender with options of 'male', 'female' and 'other', as well as religion and age. The questionnaire aimed to ascertain the participants' general knowledge of HIV, including whether they had ever obtained information about HIV and, if so, from which sources. There were more detailed questions designed to address participants' knowledge of HIV transmission, by asking whether people could get HIV in 14 possible ways, such as kissing, tattoos, breast-feeding and by sexual intercourse. The survey also asked participants whether they knew if HIV infection could be prevented and if so how, with six possible ways stipulated, including avoiding drug taking, condom use during sexual intercourse and not sharing needles.

Data Collection, Entry and Analysis

Data were collected in paper questionnaire form and manually entered into an SPSS computer package by the researcher; each survey that was entered was checked again for discrepancies. The same researcher (SB) entered the data from all 252 surveys.

The original data set had 58 variables but for some questions a new variable was created using Excel to count the numbers that correctly answered the question, essentially creating a new tool for correctness. This served to make the assessing of 'correct' knowledge about HIV transmission and prevention easier. SPSS statistical analysis was performed including chi-squared testing to test for any significant differences between the responses of different groups of participants.

References

Bloor, M., & Wood, F. (2006). *Keywords in qualitative methods: A vocabulary of research concepts.* London: Sage.

Glaser, B. G., & Strauss, A. L. (1967). *The discovery of grounded theory: Strategies for qualitative research.* Chicago: Aldine.

Ling, T. (2006). *Using qualitative methods. Oxford handbook of public health practice.* Oxford: Oxford University Press.

Nije-Carr, V. (2009). Knowledge, attitudes, cultural, social and spiritual beliefs on health seeking behaviours of Gambian adults with HIV/AIDS. *International Journal of Cultural Mental Health, 2*(2), 18–128.

Pope, C., Ziebland, S., & Mays, N. (2000). Qualitative research in health care: Analysing qualitative data. *British Medical Journal, 320,* 114–116.

Wong, L. P., Leng Chin, C. K., Low, W. Y., & Jaafar, N. (2008). HIV/AIDS knowledge among Malaysian young adults: Findings from a nationwide survey. *Medscape Journal of Medicine, 10*(6), 148.

Zou, J., Yamanaka, Y., John, M., Watt, M., Ostermann, J., & Thielman, N. (2009). Religion and HIV in Tanzania: Influence of religious beliefs on HIV stigma, disclosure, and treatment attitudes. *BMC Public Health, 9,* 75.

Chapter 4
Findings

Qualitative Results

In-depth analysis of the 35 transcripts identified the following ten central themes with associated sub-themes:

1. Islam's view of life, health and wellbeing
2. Knowledge about HIV
3. Sex outside marriage
4. Current HIV prevention in Malaysia
5. Condoms
6. Transgender women
7. Men who have Sex with Men
8. Law and authority
9. Stakeholder relationships
10. Action to be taken by stakeholders.

The qualitative findings are discussed here within each of these ten themes.

Islam's View of Life, Health and Wellbeing

Throughout the course of the interviews, participants expressed the importance of Islam for their lives, in how they conduct themselves and how they view life itself. The influence of Islam was seen as permeating one's daily life, choices, behaviours and ways of viewing the world:

© The Author(s) 2018
S. Barmania, M.J. Reiss, *Islam and Health Policies Related
to HIV Prevention in Malaysia*, SpringerBriefs in Public Health,
https://doi.org/10.1007/978-3-319-68909-8_4

Islam is also about how one conducts his or her everyday activities and this goes beyond
prayers, fasting ... it involves things like how you deal with other people, how you do busi-
ness ... (1, Religious Leader)[1]

Islam was perceived as something all encompassing, holistic and quite different
to the concept of religion in the West which is often thought of as private, secular
and wholly differentiated from public life:

Islam is not a religion in the western sense of the word ... it's a way of life ... It covers
everything I guess from the birth till the death. (35, Religious Leader)

This sentiment is often expressed by Muslims in both the Muslim and non-
Muslim world by the assertion that 'Islam is not just a religion; it's a way of life' and
thus this statement was an entry point for discussion to elicit opinion amongst the
stakeholders. Most of the participants' responses confirmed that this was an applicable statement that articulated the pivotal role Islam had on their lifecycle. This
was reiterated across the different stakeholders interviewed, not just by religious
leaders, whom one might expect to share such a standpoint, but also from the
Ministry of Health and from those within the community of PLHIV, including those
from the MSM community:

Islam actually for me ... is a way of life ... is a way of your direction towards how you live
everyday, what you always do and it's a relationship between you and God. (22, PLHIV
MSM)

However, there is an acceptance that simply following the rules may be more
difficult than one would like and that society has to accept the reality that not all
Muslims behave in exact accordance with the prescribed rules set down by the
Qur'an:

That means for the Muslim ... we must follow [the rules] but sometimes we are human,
I think we choose the wrong road sometimes ... (6, PLHIV Transgender Woman)

The idea that humans are fallible appears in various guises throughout the interviews, often intertwined with the contradiction of the ideal of how a Muslim ought
to be behaving compared with actuality. These rules are seen as a spiritual duty to
obey God (*Allah*) but also as a means of protection and prevention, which included
safeguarding of one's own health:

So it means that Islam is a way of life and within the religion was built in how to prevent
the disease and at the same time, if you get the disease, you have to seek treatment. (3,
Ministry of Health)

Islam and health ... you know, goes side by side. There is no, there is no contradictions. (25,
Ministry of Health)

The religious leaders interviewed placed a great importance on the virtue of
health and often referred back to Qur'anic texts or scripture during the interview:

---

[1] Interviewee identities are indicated by a number, which has no significance other than that it
remains the same for each interviewee, and their stakeholder group.

There is so much guidance given in Islam, either through the *Qur'an* or the prophetic traditions, on how Muslims should look after themselves in terms of health, in terms of diet, in terms of keeping one healthy ... (1, Religious Leader)

This guidance talked not only about the onus of a Muslim to look for a cure for a malady, but to also prevent and take measures to guard against ill health in the first place. Interviewees had a broad definition of health, not only restricted to the human body or mind but also encompassing the soul. There was not a clear delineation between matters that were considered of the spiritual domain and those that were physical matters. The following extract expresses this holistic attitude to health succinctly and often aspects of this were indicated in interviews with other participants:

This is the holistic way of understanding the human being, understanding all the dimensions of being human so the health of the material aspect will be taken care of, in doing all the empirical things that take care of the body of the human being but that was not separated from the other aspect of his health which is his mental health...his spiritual health ... And then they are all together in one approach towards the health of this creature who is the human being. (35, Religious Leader)

This was echoed by other stakeholders, namely officials of the Ministry of Health, who felt that health was not limited to the individual person but extended to a collective mass of people that constitute the Muslim *ummah*:

Health of the *ummah* is sustained. (10, Ministry of Health)

In many ways, this is essentially the main paradigm of modern day public health schools of thought—treating populations not just individuals.

The whole *Qur'an* is a way of preventing harm in a wider sense ... whether to body or society as a whole. (25, Ministry of Health)

As a Muslim, we have to prevent ourself from any harm. (12, Religious Leader)

However, in reality, situations are far more complex and participants were aware that there was often more than one specific 'harm' facing an individual, population or society; there were a myriad of potential harms. In such situations, the concept of adopting the principle of 'lesser harm', prioritizing the prevention of one harm over another was mentioned by participants. A few religious leaders interviewed did discuss the possibility of utilising the Islamic jurisprudence (*fiqh*) of lesser harm (*darar*) in certain situations or contexts but this was certainly not the archetypal response from imams but a minority view:

I think you need to look at the menace, the evil that you are facing and there are certain religious, legal maxims and principles ... two evils and you do not have an exit, a way out. You have to accept one at the expense of the other lesser evil. (9, Religious Leader)

Utilising 'lesser evil' was seen as a *bona fide* option by a minority of participants in circumstances where simply choosing to take no action at all would be detrimental. However, this was only mentioned by a couple of religious leader who lay along the more progressive spectrum of Islamic religious leadership and were also among the most highly educated. The use of this principle seemed to depend on people's understanding of Islamic jurisprudence. A few participants mentioned

that sometimes a person has to use his own independent judgement, a concept
known as *isthihad*:

> Then I am going to practise my independent judgement based on *ishtihad* ... *isthihad* is to
> take whatever the surrounding of that matter into the conclusion. (24, Religious Leader)

The use of *ishtihad* was not a typical response but has been mentioned by some
progressive religious leaders as a way of tackling modern day problems which perhaps were not explicitly mentioned in the *Qur'an* and *Sunnah*:

> ... and in certain circumstance, we go beyond the four schools [of thought], on the basis of
> *maslaha*; what is the interest for the public or for the country. (24, Religious Leader)

> Islam as a matter of as we mentioned, way of life recognises the local custom. Local custom
> is very important ... Islam as a religion and local customs has to be mixed; you cannot get
> rid of that. (24, Religious Leader)

The four schools of thought reflected the geographical locations of Islam and
understood that culture and context are important. This idea of independent judgement and that people can perhaps respectfully enquire about specific aspects of
Islam depending on the circumstance was raised, for example in the case of fasting
for those infected with HIV:

> But to me, it [Islam] can be challenged on certain point ... based on your needs, based on
> your types of life. (18, PLHIV MSM)

The issue of fasting whilst HIV positive posed a predicament for a number of
people living with HIV and is pertinent as it illustrates the potential conflict between
doing the best for one's health and the best for one's religion. Although some
believed that interpretations of Islam allowed for this reconciling between the two,
there was fear of what people would think and a self-propagated peer pressure of
sorts. The scenario mentioned in the excerpt above is an example of a very specific
problem of how choices that can have consequences on health are affected by religion. In Islam it is widely acknowledged that if you are unfit or medically unwell
you are granted omission from fasting or pay a charitable amount to avoid fasting;
however, there was the added pressure of worrying what the Muslim community
would think of them if they were either known to not be fasting or if they were seen
to be breaking a fictitious fast.

This dilemma is set within a context of the Islamic principle of not exposing the
sin, whereby a person should not expose the sins of others, which can create a pre-
carious balance between not exposing the 'sin' and complete denial of the 'sin', as
mentioned by one participant:

> Cover the sins, you must cover the sins, you must cover the sins and you have reward from
> *Allah*. (33, Religious Leader)

There was also mentioning by participants that although a part of Islam was the
following of rules, another element of Islam was the wholehearted belief that *Allah*
is the most merciful and forgives our shortcomings.

Knowledge About HIV

All the participants interviewed had some awareness of the existence of HIV, but the extent of their knowledge of the disease varied considerably. There was a general perception from PLHIV that there was not enough openness about the disease because it was associated with negative activities:

I think Islam is not too open about this disease, because when we talk about HIV they see we do a wrong thing, we do free sex, we do action and a bad thing. (26, PLHIV MSM)

There was a strong sense of denial, stigma and discrimination and inaccurate information:

Most people seem to be in a state of denial and they think that as long as it doesn't happen to me or my family, it's not my problem. (1, Religious Leader)

There were stout connotations of being HIV positive being associated with simply mentioning 'HIV', and of perceptions which were already preformed:

They say you have HIV, so you have no future. (12, Religious Leader)

All participants interviewed had at least some information about how HIV was transmitted, with the majority of participants believing HIV was transmitted through sexual activity or intravenous drug use:

The HIV is spread from sexual act or injection ... That's the only two ways; there is no more ways. (12, Religious Leader)

Often participants could only recall that HIV was transmitted through drug use or through sexual activity, but within the PLHIV community other methods of transmission were identified:

Sex, then drugs and breast feed, and then what else? Hmmm, sharing needle, yeah. (21, PLHIV)

Often, in articulating the routes of HIV transmission, there were strong negative overtones of moral judgement intertwined and the perception that you would not acquire HIV if you were considered to be socially 'good':

If you are HIV positive means something to do with drug abuse, it can be from the drug abuse or you have unprotected sexual intercourse with different partners. (24, Religious Leader)

While many participants did have a rudimentary understanding about HIV, many PLHIV only knew about HIV upon actual diagnosis.

After she [translated via a friend] getting the disease, then only she know about HIV. She don't bother about this disease. Oh, before this she had heard the word HIV but she think she won't get the sick, so she doesn't bother. (28, PLHIV)

A particularly poignant case was that of an 18 year-old female participant who was two months pregnant and had already been HIV positive for 2 years. Before her diagnosis "she never heard" anything about HIV as was living in a more rural area and had stopped schooling at 9 years old:

> She really feel surprised and scared and afraid and she never tell about the sickness to the family; she scared. (30, PLHIV)

This was a highly atypical case, but still important as most children do attend school and thus education about HIV during academic interactions is a crucial entry point. Nevertheless, what is typical is that many of those people living with HIV had understandably increased their knowledge of the disease and prevention thereof after their diagnosis. This represents a missed opportunity to provide information about HIV prevention to the general public as well as those who are identified as high risk such as sex workers or men who have sex with men:

> She has zero information; about condom ... normal customers she will use condoms but if the customer is, as she said, handsome, macho, so she would forget the condom. (6, PLHIV Transgender Woman)

> She went through a lot of workshops which has been organised by some NGOs; now she is very confident; she knows about the prevention, not only HIV and AIDS. She also knows about STI, Sexually Transmitted Diseases like syphilis and everything, she has the confidence to go and visit the friends who are HIV positive. (6, PLHIV Transgender Woman)

This disappointment that they did not possess the adequate knowledge to prevent themselves acquiring HIV was articulated by a few participants:

> Only they got information if they come to the centres once they are diagnosed. If she knew about the usage of condoms earlier, and all this sickness, she wouldn't be in this situation. (4, PLHIV Transgender Woman)

Many acquired information on HIV through their informal networks of friends and peers and these, as well as NGOs operating in the area, constituted a key portal for disseminating information, printed material and literature was found within newspapers and magazines. Whilst others, especially adolescents and youth, had a tendency to acquire information through the internet and social media. School or university was not considered somewhere where one could be provided with information, and increasingly new media and the internet were filling the gap and compensating for this shortfall:

> So from the internet, they get the information from there. (19, PLHIV)

> No. We did not have any exposure about these things in school. From internet, not from schools, we didn't have the exposure from our school. (28, PLHIV MSM)

In addition, many of those PLHIV interviewed found NGOs to be a beneficial information source, acting as a hub:

> So in Kuala Lumpur, we have many NGOs in Kuala Lumpur. They are supporting us, like they do they give moral support. They tell us what is HIV, how to live, how to how to live with HIV in healthy way. (26, PLHIV)

A fringe information source cited by one of the conservative religious leaders was that of prominent psychologist Malik Badri, who had previously described HIV as 'the wrath of God' (35, Religious Leader). This was an atypical viewpoint as most participants were less judgemental of PLHIV but it does represent one perspective which is important to note as religious leaders do have influence.

With regards to HIV testing, some participants mentioned hesitation towards being tested due to fears of a lack of confidentiality and anonymity:

> Some of them may think that if they come to this test, their status may get leaked or people may know about their status ... (19, PLHIV)

Those who were diagnosed as HIV positive found it to be a pivotal moment in their lives and was a cause for devastation:

> She ran a lot. She was having a luxury life. Once she is sick, that is where she found out who are her friends ... who are the friends who really wants to help her. When she was in the hospital, she realised a lot of things, even she tried to commit suicide...When she was admitted in the hospital, she tried to kill herself twice. Once with IV drip, she tried to strangle herself. Second, they tied her, let her go and then she tried to jump from the window. They tied her back. She was paralysed for two months. (6, PLHIV Transgender Woman)

The new diagnosis of having a positive HIV status was often accompanied by fear, isolation and shame:

> I am really scared you know ... that I have the virus inside me ... I don't know how to explain to them ... I don't want to be alone. (20, PLHIV MSM)

Participants who were living with HIV typically would have high levels of secrecy, opting to disclose to some family members and not others; often the shame felt by them extended to the immediate family rather than being restricted to the infected individual:

> She feels very ashamed that she is sick ... Because of family's name. (6, PLHIV Transgender Woman)

Nevertheless, there was a burgeoning sentiment that attitudes needed to change and that although NGOs can fight the stigma and discrimination on behalf of those with HIV, ultimately those with HIV have to have a 'brave heart' and be open about their status to encourage others to come forward and to change societal perceptions. Through the course of the interviews it was apparent that the key issue was the cause of HIV transmission and that the disease was inextricably associated with conduct that was categorically not acceptable, such as sex outside marriage, and thus seen as a direct consequence of sinful behaviour:

> ... but because of the misconception and looking into the HIV as a sin ... it's a product of sinful action right? Wrong people, wrong doing people and that's why the magnitude of stigma and discrimination is really very huge in Malaysia. (31, Ministry of Health)

Many of the religious leaders who participated in the study stated that they believed that HIV was either a punishment from God for not following the rules or that the disease acted as a deterrent to being gay. Notwithstanding this, those that who acquired HIV through 'non-sinful' action were not seen in the same negative light as those who acquired HIV through unacceptable sexual behaviour, with those in the former group being depicted as innocent victims, for example, housewives who had been infected by their husbands. For those who were 'innocently' infected with HIV, there existed a great deal of sympathy and understanding; this is signifi-cant as it shows the primary cause of the stigma is the means by which you acquired HIV, whether through sinful or non-sinful actions. This is a clear indication of how people living with HIV are depicted; essentially, acquiring HIV is a symptom of living an immoral life and not following Islam:

> Oh I am positive, should I treat this as a sin being given by God or should I treat this as a reminder for me to have a good health? (18, PLHIV MSM)

There was also the quite open mentioning by some religious leaders that HIV was the direct result of the nefarious influence of westernisation, globalisation and the idea of 'free sex' (34, Religious Leader):

> … Malaysia is just like all the societies that have been influenced by westernisation. (35, Religious Leader)

Often the term 'free sex' was used by participants to describe their perception of sexual practices in the West. Religious leaders at the more conservative end of the spectrum were unwavering in their perception of the cause of HIV being immorality:

> … if you respect the rules and regulations that governs human sexuality, such a disease would not actually happen It's inconceivable that if people are adhering to the rules and regulations which are prescribed by the *Sharia* regarding the human sexuality, something like this will never happen. (35, Religious Leader)

Ultimately, many of the negative perceptions of those living with HIV are, to a certain degree, in some way related or arise due to the attitudes and beliefs about sex outside the confines of marriage, the importance placed on abiding by this funda-mental principle and the consequence of not doing so.

Sex Outside Marriage

The participants were quite forthcoming in expressing their attitudes towards sex in general and this was noticed across the stakeholders. There was no expectation that Muslims were to be celibate, with one religious leader saying that Islam had a more realistic and tolerant view of sex, that unlike other religions, such as Christianity, which may see sex only as a means to procreate, Islam considers sex to be an enjoy-able and permitted part of life:

> Basically procreation; it's also a recreation. (8, Religious Leader)

Furthermore, even the most conservative of religious leaders were keen to explain that historically in Islam, the Prophet (peace be upon him) had been forthright in discussing personal matters such as sex, if and when the need arose:

> These are the human activities but *Sharia* wanted these activities actually to be governed by the rules and regulations which will protect and preserve the human progeny, that's all. (35, Religious Leader)

The same participant was keen to highlight that although there is a Western modern day paradigm of sex education, the earlier Islamic literature did discuss issues regarding sex—acts that should and should not be done, personal hygiene before and after sex in a very practical sense without embarrassment or inhibition. In particular, amongst the religious leaders there was an understanding of the importance of sex as a facet of human nature, a desire created by God and one that is wholly encouraged but within limits, which are clearly prescribed. These boundaries are clearly defined—within marriage between a woman and a man, husband and wife.

> OK, to me, as far as I am concerned, any sexual relationship outside the confines of marriage *haram*, it's *haram*. (1, Religious Leader)

This was a belief expressed particularly vociferously by religious leaders along the progressive/conservative spectrum:

> Sex before marriage, I don't agree. 100 percent I don't agree. (34, Religious Leader)

In addition, across the stakeholders, including people living with HIV, MSM and people who were transgender, there was little dispute with the assertion that sex outside marriage was 'not moral' (28, PLHIV). The perception of sex outside marriage in Islamic theory was clearly *haram*; indeed, this word was reiterated throughout the interviews, especially by religious leaders, and emphasized the gravity of the act. This was also articulated from those within the medical profession, amongst the Ministry of Health:

> There is no sex outside marriage. So if anybody wants to say that how condom is permissible, *Qur'an* quote permissible outside marriage in Islam, I find that hard to swallow because as a principle, there is no sex outside marriage in Islam, so how can you bend something, bend by words ... can you want to prevent something which is not right? (25, Ministry of Health)

The excerpt above clearly reflects the difficult position that Ministry of Health officials are in; they obviously do not like people reinterpreting Islam or, as they say, 'bend[ing] by words', by suggesting that something which is not permissible is allowed. This also highlights the core sensitivity by which there may be conflicts with various stakeholders about how to prevent HIV infections. Some participants commented on both the short- and long-term consequences of sex outside marriage, not just to the individual or the religion, but also on wider society and the community, including very specific issues such as the identification of the father of the child, if the woman became pregnant, as well as legal and social security issues, such as inheritance under Islamic law. Despite this, there was discussion by many participants about the gulf that existed between the ideal of abstinence of sex before marriage (and outside marriage) versus the reality that many people including Muslims in Malaysia were unable to abide by these rules:

> Of course in Malaysia without marriage it's *haram*. You cannot but here it's natural, especially for teenagers. Have a feeling to try ... sex is something needed ... So we can't deny their human needs. (27, PLHIV)

Some participants believed there was a dichotomy between the ideal of what Malay Muslims should be doing according to Islam and societal expectations and what they were actually doing. Participants, especially from within the PLHIV community, understood the fact that there was mounting opportunity, peer pressure and a wish to experiment that made the ideal of sex only within marriage harder to adhere to:

> The teenager want to try something. (27, PLHIV)

Issues such as those described above were a concern amongst the younger generation who have grown up in the era of widespread internet access and social media and were less protected from external influences both nationally and internationally. In contrast, some of the religious leaders had the view that premarital sex could be stopped. However, other participants understood that preventing sex amongst the young would be difficult in Malaysia where education and the work environment are not segregated by gender, like in certain other parts of the Muslim world, and thus would make it harder to 'control' such activity:

> You know we can't control the youngsters because in Malaysia, we are very liberal in the sense you can mix up girls and boys, other Muslim countries where you have separation. (24, Religious leader)

There is the sentiment amongst some of the participants, especially from the PLHIV group, that some Malaysian religious leaders are fighting against a rising tide and it was simply not feasible to block premarital sex; thus, some of the NGOs are willing to provide condoms. While some couples may want to have sex but feel they are not ready to marry the opposite is also true, with some couples wanting to get married but not currently being in a financially stable enough position to be able to do so or facing parental disapproval of the marriage:

> Still now they have sex but they won't marry- no money, no job. She is working and gives him money. (29 PLHIV, Female Sex Worker)

There were many participants who felt that some stakeholders were in a state of denial:

> General stakeholder of Malaysia, they deny it that sex doesn't happen on there ... the stakeholder says that sex only happen when you are getting married ... but sex happen even as a young as twelve. (18, PHIV MSM)

Sex Education

Given that endeavouring to curb the practice of sex outside marriage seems to some to be futile, impractical or largely fraught with difficulties, one might presume that sex education, in some guise, would be implemented or at least encouraged in Malaysia. However, this is not the case. Sex education was seen as a very divisive issue because it is often perceived not only as accepting that there is a problem in the first place but also as promoting sex outside marriage:

> Yeah, I think they [religious leaders] believe that sex education is a kind of vehicle of promoting as I say, promiscuity and of promoting free sex in society, it's not about prevention, it's not about prevention of HIV. (8, Religious Leader)

The religious leaders interviewed were often strongly opposed to sex education for a multitude of reasons, including deeming its introduction as unnecessary and possibly corrupting. They often felt deeply uncomfortable with the idea of 'safe sex' which is how they interpreted sex education and their idea of an appropriate sex education curriculum would be consistent with Islamic rules of abstinence until marriage:

Abstinence is the best, OK ... They have to avoid *zina*, abstinence is still the best. Just get married. (2, Religious Leader)

Most religious leaders thought that sex education was simply not necessary, but others explained that hesitance about sex education was an attempt to prevent an open and honest discussion about sex education. There was also a genuine suspicion that sex education was a ploy to promote the Western agenda and ideals:

People think this is western agenda to talk about sex education ... to propagate free sex. (8, Religious Leader)

The views expressed by other stakeholders, the hesitation and reasons for and against sex education, were more complicated; one participant questioned who has responsibility for the sex education of children and adolescents, presenting the atypical viewpoint that overall it was the duty of the parents:

I think the parents must educate the kids and this is not taboo, it's something natural. In Islam also in itself ... in Islam have a lesson for sex but with guidance. (27, PLHIV)

While other participants were cognisant that talking about such matters in Malaysia may be beneficial, they also realised that there is a difficult balance to be struck between teaching adolescents about how best to protect themselves whilst also reconciling concern that such open discussions may be a catalyst for triggering sexual exploration. Participants from the Ministry of Health had an interesting position, focussing less on the necessity or futility of sex education and more on how to tentatively impart knowledge about prevention:

We didn't call it sex education modules. This is the health module, these are health modules. Yeah. This is not called sex education. This way people ask us, we say we don't have the sex education module. (3, Ministry of Health)

The Ministry of Health was unclear what was included in the sex education package and cautious about the terminology used, avoiding the use of the expression 'sex education' which conjured up negative connotations of 'free sex' amongst other stakeholders, such as religious leaders and within the community.

Current HIV Prevention in Malaysia

The different stakeholder groups held diverse opinions regarding past and present HIV prevention policies in Malaysia, how they have progressed so far and future directions. Particularly noticeable differences amongst stakeholders were regarding specific measures, such as condom distribution:

> Well it's been very uneven I think … the prevention policies in Malaysia. In the early days, when HIV was first detected; in the '80s, actually they were very practical and there were posters and stuff that talked about condoms and openly talked about safe sex, behaviour etc. and drugs of course; it was only later on that somehow somewhere someone kind of clamped down on some of this information. (23, PLHIV)

Many participants believed that although progress had been made the social and political climate in Malaysia made it very difficult to impose certain measures:

> Think there is a long way to prevention of HIV/AIDS in Malaysia and mostly for the Muslim communities. Because we cannot help because their religious obligations and their health obligations; it's a different thing. (14, PLHIV)

> Just to do simple practical public health things … it's very, very hard in this country. (23, PLHIV)

It was considered difficult terrain to have such discussions and implement certain policies, a constant cause of disagreement, whilst some participants were more positive towards the prevention policies, mentioning the work done on drug replacement as an example of good practice:

> I think we have done quite well in drug-related transmission, particularly our syringe replacement … That's a real success. I mean you can see the numbers really dropped. And access is quite good. (11, Ministry of Health)

The harm reduction polices aimed at preventing transmission of HIV amongst intravenous drug users was often named as policy to be proud of, across all stakeholders:

> Currently, right now they are doing quite well, in a programme what they call as NSEP, Needle Syringe Exchange Programme. (22, PLHIV MSM)

Condom Distribution

Condom distribution was often cited by all stakeholders as a prevention policy, but the opinions about this varied and it was considered a contentious issue; some participants believed that condom distribution was an acceptable practice but that access was difficult due to public opinion:

> Actually we have free condom campaign but our…our people in Malaysia can't accept the campaign because they say we are Malaysian countries, Muslim countries. (21, PLHIV)

The concern was partly about what the predominantly Muslim Malay population would think about condoms; hence condom distribution was not heavily publicised. There were differing opinions as to which bodies or organisations were distributing condoms, with many PLHIV believing that it was only distributed by themselves and not by the Ministry of Health:

> It's only obviously only done by NGOs and it's not publicised. (23, PLHIV)

Contrarily, the Ministry of Health said that condoms were available through its organisation but this was clearly a contentious issue as they received criticism from both the general public and religious leaders:

And then, when you are doing preventive measures like distribution of condoms, of course there are people who look at it from moral issues; that by so doing you are promoting free sex. (11, Ministry of Health)

However, the Ministry of Health had tried to reframe the problem by changing the language, favouring 'disease prevention', to reassert that HIV prevention was a public health issue:

We are looking at disease control mechanism, keeping away from the moral components of it. So we just look at it as health workers; this is the disease control; there is a disease, it's spread through this, so as a control mechanism. (11, Ministry of Health)

Premarital HIV Testing

Another HIV prevention strategy mentioned by participants was the premarital HIV testing policy for Muslim Malay couples. The history of the policy is particularly interesting, as it was implemented gradually before it was employed across the country, as described by the following participant:

It was started in 2001, in the state of Johor. And after that it started scaling up in others [states] I mean, it spread in other states and now almost every state has the programme on pre-marital screening. (3, Ministry of Health)

Participants, for the most part, perceived premarital HIV testing to be a positive venture:

This is good [pre-marital HIV testing] … to protect. (33, Religious Leader)

One participant, a middle-aged housewife living with HIV, who had contracted the disease from her husband, had the belief that perhaps it could have prevented her case if she had had the test:

OK, she never do the test. She say it's very good from getting the awareness. (28, PLHIV)

Opponents of pre-marital HIV testing in general have argued that such measures could be used for nefarious purposes, criminalising or at least stigmatising those living with HIV. However, the support for premarital testing was considerable, specifically amongst religious leaders who participated in the study and who considered that it was providing a protective mechanism, in line with the teachings of the *Sharia*, and was not criminalising or stigmatising:

Well I think the *Sharia* would like to protect people against any kind of harm. So in that regard, I think right step to be taken. No it's not criminalising anybody but the *Sharia* would like to protect the individual, *hukm*. (35, Religious Leader)

It's a good idea. Of course, there are pros and cons. (25, Ministry of Health)

Some participants, including religious leaders, felt that although they fully supported premarital HIV testing as it was in line with the *hukm* (protection of life, heredity, lineage etc), there should be a degree of privacy and confidentiality. However, where exactly the boundaries of privacy and confidentiality should be drawn remained unclear as some believed that since a marital union in Islam is the joining of two families, both families and the imam should know the HIV status of each person tested, whilst others believed that it was up to the individual to disclose their status to whom they wish:

Some participants were unsure as to which stakeholder requested pre-marital HIV testing in Malaysia, with the consensus believing that it was instigated by religious leaders:

> Pre-marital screening test, I was directly involved in it, in this project...when we were discussing with the religious department...the idea of the pre-marital screening came from the religious department of Johor, from the mufti himself, looking at the issue of HIV among Muslim in Johor during, I think 2000-2001. So he felt that the Muslim leadership come down and reach those people who are at risk of getting HIV. So it was the religious initiative. And we supported that. (31, Ministry of Health)

Initialised by religious leaders to be taken up by Muslims, the premarital test is now offered to non-Muslims and is now normalised in Malaysian society. Nevertheless, there has been an issue as to whether the testing is a legal requirement for Muslims or not and whether it's mandatory or voluntary. The following excerpt highlights the conflicting sentiments expressed by the one individual in the Ministry of Health:

> That's done actually mainly for Muslim couples. For the non-Muslims it's not compulsory because there are different perspectives of it. But again, HIV screening has always been voluntary. So they have made it mandatory for other things, so there is this issue of whether it should be made a legal requirement and all but as it is the decision of the Muslim council, then all those Muslims couples who have to marry have to undergo that. (11, Ministry of Health).

The pre-marital HIV test was seen as both cost effective and a good form of prevention, including the prevention of social and marital disharmony:

> Prevention of social disharmony or social, to prevent marriage disharmony, I believe it's very cost effective. (25, Ministry of Health)

The language is used to articulate a message in a more accepting way, so although testing is not obligatory under the Ministry of Health, it is obligatory under the Ministry of Religious Affairs if you wish to marry and this testing service is under the remit of the Ministry of Health. However, there are elements that suggest that although the Ministry of Health agree with such testing, they also express some concerns and can exert a certain amount of influence:

> So based on the religious decree they put it as compulsory. But we said that OK, if you put it as compulsory, there should be some conditions. (31, Ministry of Health)

In this sense, the Ministry of Health has some ability to negotiate with the religious leaders to get the best 'deal' in the interest of the public. The caveat stipulated by the Ministry of Health is that with pre-marital testing there must also be pre and post-test counselling which is in accordance with standard HIV guidelines:

> But it's fine so long as they advise the couple pre-test counselling and all, they can actually adjust ... be able to adjust to the implications of the results which they might get. So that's very, very important on how they do. Otherwise there could be issues. (11, Ministry of Health)

> WHO says no you can't have mandatory premarital HIV testing ... the only way to really get this done was to go through the state religious office. (23, PLHIV)

The excerpt above is illuminating as it suggests there are outside forces of influence, in this instance the World Health Organisation, that premarital testing may not have been the idea of the Ministry of Religious Affairs but actually the Ministry of Health. The key message is that there are strong power dynamics and influence at play between the Ministry of Health and the Department of Religious Affairs.

Condoms

The issue of condom usage was contentious, with the opinions expressed by different stakeholders varied and polemical and different parties often staunchly in favour or against. Typically, participants associated condoms with sexual activity outside of marriage and thus not in keeping with the rules of Islam; this was particularly felt by religious leaders:

> People here relate condoms to free sex or sex outside marriage. (1, Religious Leader)

Even amongst those that advocated condom usage, there was a fundamental realization that at best they were viewed as forbidden, offensive and not in keeping with Malaysian values. Condoms were seen as taboo and as a promoter of 'free sex', whilst it was also realised that they had a role to play in the prevention of HIV:

> They are still taboo; condoms some can accept it, some people can't, encouraging them to have sex but no not at all. (4, PLHIV Transgender Woman)

Even carrying condoms was associated with illicit activity forbidden in Islam, such as sex work and Men who have Sex with Men. However, all religious leaders interviewed allowed for the use of condoms in serodiscordant married couples as this was understood to prevent HIV transmission to the uninfected partner:

> No, if they are married, one of them have HIV, OK we can give them condoms. (2, Religious Leader)

Extending this allowance further, to the majority, seemed by some participants as though it would expose people or make them more likely to engage in *zina*. Jabatan Kemajuan Islam Malaysia (JAKIM) were particularly against condom distribution and wanted their standpoint to be conveyed:

> This is one of our stand, JAKIM stands, not to give the condom to unmarried people. Condoms is just to the people who are married, maybe one of the spouse have infected with

HIV, so it can be done. But if they are not infected, it's very forbidden, So we are not compromising that. (2, Religious Leader)

This was at odds with those that benefitted from condoms the most, PLHIV:

For us, for PLHIV, condom is very important to use, we must accept that we have to use this condom, without condom that disease will transfer to other person. (26, PLHIV)

Most of the religious leaders thought of condoms as intrinsically *haram*, even when probed to consider the idea of greater and lesser harm; apart from under the circumstance of a couple with HIV, it was considered compiling one *haram* on top of another *haram*:

I can't accept that one, you did the *haram* thing but on top of that you have protection this is *haram* but to have protection is something better than not having that I think it is...applies in the certain circumstances and it is in this Islamic principles, some principles. (24, Religious Leader)

Amongst some of the more progressive religious leaders interviewed, there was a view that the condom itself was neutral but had the potential to be a tool for *haram* or *halal*:

For a valid purpose and I think to curb the spread of disease, lethal disease like AIDS. I accept that condom use in principle is allowed. (9, Religious Leader)

A related atypical viewpoint was that for any instrument or technology, the tool is not inherently *haram* or *halal*, but the way in which it is used and the intention of its use are the deciding factors in making it one or the other:

It's not just about condoms, or anything for that matter. I am of the opinion that whatever that you have – a tool, a technology, a gadget – it's not the thing but it is your intention. It goes back to your intention. (1, Religious Leader)

Actual condom usage in Malaysia was determined by practical issues such as personal preference, ability to negotiate condom usage, cost and awareness:

I think the awareness is high. I believe the younger generation probably are using it quite extensively, it's not a taboo I think as far as the usage of condom's concerned. Those who are active sexually, whether pre-marital or you know. (11, Ministry of Health)

No, last time I don't prefer to use condoms, I don't like it. (5, PLHIV Transgender Woman)

Some participants were well versed in the virtues of condom usage in relation to HIV prevention, especially in high risk scenarios such as sex work, but their negotiating power was limited by their customers or clients who did not wish to use them. Sex workers found themselves subject to market forces and had to forsake protection for financial remuneration, indicative of the power dynamics between the professional sex worker and the client paying for the service:

Condom is the prevention, to have safe sex ... if the customer don't use condom, she don't take the customers; if you want [sex] you have to use condoms. (7, PLHIV Transgender Woman)

Despite this, there were other participants who did feel empowered and confident enough to demand condom usage and would rather forsake the customer than the protection provided by a condom:

> She say the person won't accept the condom, she won't accept the person [translated via a friend]. (29, PLHIV Female Sex Worker)

Another barrier to condom usage was the cost relative to earnings; although available to purchase for a few ringgits, the financial costs soon multiply and often amongst female sex workers the fear of pregnancy instigated condom usage more than the threat of acquiring HIV:

> For one, three ringgit she pay, everyday she use it, every time she got customer. Sometimes the condom is soft, it's ruptured … she is scared of getting pregnant … so use always use that. (29, PLHIV)

PLHIV also cited fear, intimidation and extortion by the police authorities as further reasons for avoidance of condom usage or even carrying condoms. Even though under Malaysian law you are allowed to carry condoms, doing so risks their being used against you as circumstantial evidence, discussed in more detail under the legal system later in this chapter.

Transgender Women

The overall perception in Malaysian society of those who were transgender was decidedly negative and transgender women were considered a marginalised, vulnerable part of society. Changing one's gender was simply not recognised by religious leaders across the spectrum and all those transgender participants living with HIV who were interviewed were well aware of how they and other fellow transgender women were perceived. The transgender population was associated with illicit and criminal activities, such as sex work and drug use:

> They are equated to being sex workers. (16, PLHIV)

Other stakeholders described transgender women as a 'vehicle for transmission of sexually transmitted diseases' (8, Religious Leader).

Amongst other PLHIV there was more sympathy and appreciation that the transgender community is a highly visible and marginalised minority within society perceived as being linked to ill health and sexual activity:

> They perceive a transgender as not a healthy community and transgender is a community that will link to sexual activities like sex. (18, PLHIV MSM)

Transgender participants felt ostracised from mainstream society and experienced demonization particularly amongst religious leaders:

> Ustad [religious leader], they said LGBT they are illness; they are mental illness…For me to be successful, we cannot involve with them … They won't do anything for us. They still say haram. (5, PLHIV Transgender Woman)

There was much scepticism by the transgender community when religious leaders did make an effort to engage with them, particularly when this was accompanied by conditions, such as requiring a transgender woman to dress as a man. This was the scenario described by a transgender woman who sought help from a caseworker who facilitated her placement in a religiously run shelter house, where she had an unfavourable experience:

> She [translated via a friend] started seeking help from the caseworker this and that, but she was put in the house and that's where she started to encounter the religious people. OK? You just be a man. So that's why she cut her hair everything and ... She looks like this but her heart's still a woman ... It's because she is saying that in the house, there are certain rules and she is engaging with the religious department ... She is not comfortable in herself. (4, PLHIV Transgender Woman)

The participant explained in her interview that her attire was masculine due to the fact that the shelter home does not allow her to remain unless she dresses as a woman. Such conditions sully the relationship between the transgender community and religious leaders. These tensions are accentuated by the religious leaders running *muhayam* camps, explained later in this chapter.

The Ministry of Health has also been reaching out to the transgender community, but not explicitly with a view of converting people back to their birth gender, but more in the sense of disease control and prevention:

> But as far as our Ministry is concerned, we do reach out for them in their various groups in terms of disease control, knowing that they got certain high risk lifestyle. (11, Ministry of Health)

Nevertheless, there was often a recognition amongst the Ministry of Health that there was an underlying and perhaps unresolvable issue, that the Ministry of Health did not recognise them as transgender, as an official gender:

> That is an issue, because in the Muslim community they don't recognise that [transgender]. So when I say don't recognise them, to accept them as a legal entity and to treat the issues around, it's quite difficult. Or human talking about their rights and all those kind of thing. (11, Ministry of Health)

This is all a departure from how transgender people have historically been integrated in Malay society, for example in terms of entertainment:

> Traditionally, transgender people have been well accepted in Malay society; you will find them everywhere, you go to weddings, all the ones that do the makeup, the hair. (23, PLHIV)

However, the above represents an atypical viewpoint expressed towards the transgender community in Malaysia. The central feature is the ruling of Islam, with respect to transgenderism:

> Presenting as a woman, it's not allowed. He is a man and he presents himself as a woman, maybe from his dressing sign or his body language sign, it's not allowed. We are not permitted to change ourselves. (12, Religious Leader)

Apart from the Islamic view that men should not impersonate characteristics of women, in terms of dressing and mannerism, a further argument mentioned by this particular participant is that any change to the body, such as tattooing or cosmetic surgery is *haram*; it entails changing what has been given to you by *Allah* the Creator, who is all knowledgeable, and is harming the body given to you by God. Nevertheless, there is an appreciation that there are people who are of physically indeterminate sex, a medical condition which naturally exists in the wider population, in Muslim and other societies now and throughout history, referred to as *khunsa*:

> *Khunsa*, in Malaysia we are very strict in the Muslims scholars, the muftis, the Muslim preachers are very strict in that sense and he or she has to, to make up his mind based on both emotional and also factors of whatsoever. (24, Religious Leader)

However the guidelines for *khunsa* are strict and few in number and most of the transgender population do not fall into this category:

> We recognise *khunsa* but we do not recognise transgender. (2, Religious Leader)

Religious leaders were clear in that there was male, female and in some rare cases, *khunsa*. Some religious leaders, namely JAKIM, had developed their own specific programmes, called the *muhayam* camps, for the transgender population, by befriending them.

> We have our own programme. JAKIM have developed a programme that we call *muhayam*; *muhayam* that means camping. (2, Religious Leader)

> Cure. Information and cure. Transgender, we go to them ... transgender, we teach them this is not good. We don't say *haram*, we do not; but this is not good. Man, why do you become a woman. (2, Religious Leader)

JAKIM were clear that these camps were not 'conversion camps' as they have been labelled by the transgender community, NGOs and human rights organisations. In addition, it seems that these camps are supported, not financially but in other ways, by the Ministry of Health:

> But somehow in Islam, this issue can be corrected. I am very supportive of the ways JAKIM trying to do the *muhayam* activities, try to bring back these people to be corrected into as men or whatsoever. (3, Ministry of Health)

Such actions by JAKIM and interactions by some sectors of the religious groups, however well-intentioned, have only served to cause conflict and increase distrust within the transgender community and other stakeholders. Transgender participants who had interacted with other religious leaders felt they were greeted with condemnation and pressure to 'come back' to their birth gender and thus felt more comfortable with NGOs such as the PT Foundation where they felt 'safe':

> *Ustads*, definitely they will advise me, they will condemn me, *haram* they say, they will ask me to come back to be a male. I feel more comfortable here with PT. I feel safe. I feel safe. (5, PLHIV Transgender Woman)

The word 'safe' in the above excerpt is poignant but it is not entirely clear whether it refers to physical or emotional safety. Nevertheless, it was a word which was often heard in the interviews. It could allude to feeling morally chastised by the religious authorities and police or to more direct action, such as being fined or arrested, as mentioned by another transgender participant:

> Religious department, of course they arrest you, you have to pay this amount...And then, they will ask you to change and then they give you counselling. But what she says, whatever they do, whatever they do, they cannot change. (6, PLHIV Transgender Woman)

Most of the transgender participants interviewed had had unfavourable experiences not only with the religious people but also with the police:

> As a transgender in Malaysia, she went through a lot of risky stuff like police ... with police, religious department ... with the religious department; normally they chase them. You have to pay fine, sometimes as usual, they ask you to come back to the path ... And police will chase them. They [religious leaders] are not supportive; they are giving a lot of trouble. (7, PLHIV Transgender Woman)

Even more severe mistreatment was verbalised by some of the interviewed transgender participants, such as beating, being stripped or made to show parts of their body against their wishes:

> I think one time only, one of the officer, a police, they stopped me, they caught me ... Then they brought me to the police station ... they asked me to go once toilet, they asked me to open my backside [Laughs]. Then they beat me, they beat my backside, really. The police, so bad. Actually I begged them you know, I begged them please, I said I am a working person, I am not prostitute. (5, PLHIV Transgender Woman)

Such accounts are particularly important because they give credence to much of what the transgender community and other sources, such as Human Rights Watch, have expressed. However, religious groups and the Ministry of Health have often said that these are isolated or exaggerated events. There was also discussion of whether transgender women were able to access healthcare and what were some of the barriers to accessing treatment. One particular issue is that on their identity cards such women are defined as men, although they look like women and most feel very uncomfortable placed in male wards. Also, some participants stated that they were discriminated against by some health care professionals, not so much by doctors but by nurses.

The final result is that transgender communities are 'driven underground' and less likely to access services. Ultimately this damages HIV prevention efforts; unsurprisingly transgender individuals state that they feel more comfortable with NGOs:

> It poses huge challenges for HIV prevention work; because of the stigma and discrimination transgenders are driven underground and are afraid to come forward to access prevention and care services from mainstream providers. (32, PLHIV)

Men Who have Sex with Men (MSM)

Although members of the LGBT community are often grouped together in Malaysian society, it is crucially important to look at the subgroups separately. The perception of Men who have Sex with Men in Malay society is that they tend to be the more highly educated:

> MSM community is mostly the intelligent community. They are not homeless, they got own job, our NGO don't have any problem to give them any information about HIV they say if they have a session to talk about HIV, they always come, no problem. (26, PLHIV)

The NGOs were much better at accessing the MSM community compared to other PLHIV ones. However, there was the perception amongst many who were interviewed for the study that Men who have Sex with Men were doing so at a cost to Malay society:

> Man and man *haram* and for society it's not good. (33, Religious Leader)

Other participants were clear to differentiate between the actual physical act of anal sex between two men and the western notion of homosexuality, with the act being unacceptable. This differentiation between the act and orientation is vital. The majority of religious leaders who were interviewed had negative opinions about Men who have Sex with Men:

> Abnormal, it's disgusting, not acceptable. (35, Religious Leader)

Even those who were from the PLHIV community understood that societally it was considered wrong but also that sexuality was part of their human rights:

> It's something wrong but this is human rights. (27 PLHIV MSM)

> Gay is not a disease. (18, PLHIV MSM)

Notwithstanding such assertions, the spectre of condemnation was never too far away with most religious leaders believing that such activity constituted a "grave sin" (IV 35 religious leader). The following excerpt from a religious leader articulates the feeling amongst mainstream Islamic leaders that homosexuality is against the teachings of Islam. There is acknowledgement that homosexual activity (MSM) does exist in Malay society but one should not be promoting such actions or being too tolerant:

> Of course it is something against the teaching of Islam; it is prohibited not only in the religion of Islam, it applies to all the other religions, it happens but we don't want to have a policy encouraging these things. (24, Religious Leader)

Often, religious leaders quoted directly from the *Qur'an* and *Sunnah*, providing evidence why homosexuality is forbidden with reference to the Story of *Lut*:

> [The *Qur'an*] says that he [*Allah*] has destroyed the whole community of *Lut* because they practised these homosexual activities; that has been mentioned clearly in the *Qur'an*. (24, Religious Leader)

Those MSM interviewed were aware that their sexual action was also considered a criminal activity and related to Section 377 of the law, even though it constituted a private affair between two consenting adults, bolstering the feeling that MSM were engaged in wrongful and illegal activities:

> He's a criminal, because we do have three Acts, three sections actually; I think 377, A, B and C about being, being homosexual and being sodomised. (22, PLHIV MSM)

Although there was such a law, it seemed to many, including the MSM community itself, that this was not operationalised or enforced:

> Men who are having Sex with Men, to me is like I have seen a lot of gay around KL and none of them have been charged for the penal code [laughs]. (18, PLHIV MSM)

The law is therefore seen as 'theoretical' rather than a law which is enforced, with participants, even those who supposedly could be prosecuted under it, finding it paradoxical and nonsensical that the law still existed when it was very rarely used; across stakeholders there was agreement that the law rarely led to convictions of sodomy. Some participants, mainly from the PLHIV community, believed that the law, though archaic, should be repealed, as the existence of such a law serves to create a disabling and stigmatising environment for HIV prevention. On the other hand those interviewed from the Ministry of Health mostly believed the law was not a deterrent or affected the lives of MSM:

> So for that purpose, the law is there but I have not seen many cases in which people have been charged. (11, Ministry of Health)

Other participants expressed the belief that the law's existence was a political tool which could then be manipulated for corruption:

> In the Malaysian context, it's completely tied up with politics ... the atmosphere really has gotten much more difficult because of politics. (23, PLHIV)

The usage of the word 'sodomy' is somewhat peculiar; it is an anachronistic term, implying moral judgement and its use is considered inappropriate in the mainstream HIV arena. It is worth noting that the word also has religious connotations in Judaeo-Christianity as well as within Islam, owing to the story of Sodom and Gomorrah in *Genesis*. Participants from the MSM community did not see it as a choice to be homosexual but a deeply imbedded part of their nature, yet they were acutely aware that being gay was against the cultural, religious and social norms of Malaysia:

> We can't do that because that is the rules and regulations. We can't do that actually because it is against our religion. (21, PLHIV MSM)

This is a very typical response by people in the MSM category, that essentially their sexuality was not a choice, whilst other stakeholders disagreed. The majority of the MSM interviewed feel that actively being gay as well as Muslim was not a contradiction: they compartmentalized the two areas of their lives: their spiritual, religious selves and their sexual lives:

> Even he is gay, he is still fasting, he is still five times prayer per day – he is still gay. (18, PLHIV MSM)

Whilst some MSM felt they could not speak to Islamic religious leaders because they were judgemental, others felt that some religious leaders were more approachable:

> Depends on that person itself because some of them are very supportive but some of them are very judgemental. (21, PLHIV MSM)

Some of the religious leaders interviewed felt that the best solution for MSM was that they should get married to a woman:

> Woman is for the protection, protection and forget their desire. (33, Religious Leader)

Amongst the MSM PLHIV community, some participants expressed concern at the growing number of those being diagnosed with HIV but did not feel that this affected access to treatment:

> In terms of gay life, umm, access to treatment, there is no such problem so far, it's just that, it becomes so obvious in a hospital right now, out of ten of all community seven is MSM positive attended and it becomes a big population now. (18, PLHIV MSM)

Many in the MSM community were married (to women) and this constituted a definite problem in terms of access to HIV prevention services as they were hesitant to access appropriate information:

> It's quite difficult because they are quite discreet and they didn't want people know that they are MSM and it's hard for us to give information on how to prevent themselves. (19, PLHIV MSM)

Some of these factors of not wanting to disclose sexuality due to being married or religious or because of societal condemnation made access to HIV prevention services difficult and drove the community underground, essentially resulting in them being hard to reach. Even amongst participants from the Ministry of Health it was acknowledged that MSM (and also the transgender community) in Malaysia are a hard to reach group and thus having contacts such as those within the NGO community is vital if health providers are to disseminate information and services relating to HIV:

> Homosexuals OK, very hard to reach. Of course, I must admit that you know, having contacts is very important, contacts with the communities, transgender communities, homosexual communities, is very important. (25, Ministry of Health)

Law and Authority

The subject of law, authority and human rights presented itself in various guises through the course of the interviews with the participants. Issues pertaining to criminal law in Malaysia as well as Islamic *Sharia* law were raised. Section 377, the Article in law relating to acts of sodomy, was mentioned by a minority of participants, mainly from within the PLHIV community, who disagreed with the existence of such a law, whilst also conceding that in Malaysia this would be highly unlikely to be changed:

I think the law in Malaysia is quite nonsense because people are doing it in reality [referring to MSM]. (19, PLHIV)

Although the laws exist this did not prevent illegal acts, such as sex work, occurring; however, there was a need to access these marginalised groups:

Because prostitution as such, I mean professional sex workers; it's illegal in this country, but yet, we have to reach out, right? (11, Ministry of Health)

In this excerpt, the participant from the Ministry of Health is self-correcting their language in line with language that is more acceptable in the international HIV arena. They also mentioned that some laws were confusing and presumed that women were sex workers by having condoms in their possession, which was not seen favourably by many within the PLHIV community:

We also have a lot of other things, you know, stupid laws like if women are found with condoms in their handbags, they are assumed to be soliciting. (23, PLHIV)

Islamic, *Sharia* law was also mentioned in relation to cross dressing, *liwat* (men who have sex with men and *khalwat*, the idea of 'close proximity' between two people of the opposite gender. Although these matters (apart from public cross dressing) may involve the private domain of individual households, many of the religious leaders felt these issues were part of the wider *Sharia* of how to govern oneself, the country and the Muslim *ummah*, thus were deemed as public matters. However, one participant atypically questioned this viewpoint by reaffirming the principle in Islam of respecting the privacy of others:

Islam doesn't permit the people to invade the privacy of others. (8, Religious Leader)

There was an unresolved debate between differing stakeholders as to whether the current laws in Malaysia were interfering with HIV prevention in the country and whether they should, or rather could, be changed or modified in some way. All participants from the Ministry of Health had the viewpoint that the laws would not change and that such discussions were futile. There was also a sense that they felt pressured in some way to justify the laws, which were not part of their mandate as the Ministry of Health, but as they represent the government, they felt they were questioned on this. The following series of excerpts from one member of the Ministry of Health is typical of the thoughts and views of all those from the Ministry who participated in the study:

People keep asking why can't the government change the law. It's not an easy process. What our aim here is to look into the activity that able for us to get an impact for the people. (3, Ministry of Health)

The prime argument of the Ministry of Health was that these laws did not have an effect on the work they were practically able to do in preventing HIV, with one participant citing laws surrounding drug use:

For example, is there any change in law regarding drugs? Do they change a single word in the law, are we able to penetrate to do some activities on harm reductions? So law is still there but sometimes it's needed but somehow we do some works ... Change the law? You are wasting your time, because you must understand that law is being made in Parliament. (3, Ministry of Health)

Notwithstanding this, many of those from the PLHIV community believed that the current laws should be changed and that their existence hampers HIV prevention by facilitating corruption by those who enforce the laws, i.e. the police officers:

It all lends itself a lot, to a lot of corruption, I want to get off, OK I will pay you. (23, PLHIV)

Human Rights

In many Western societies, the concept of human rights is one that is held by many people to be absolute, and maintaining these values is considered essential. However, in Malaysia, the notion of human rights has been controversial and in this research differing views of its importance were held by the various stakeholder groups; indeed interviewees in the Ministry of Health were careful not to engage in discussion on human rights. All in all, human rights were not considered universal as they are generally regarded in the western world, because there are other features such as the rule of law and religious values that govern the country and that there are occasions where these latter values take precedence over notions of human rights. This issue of rights came to the fore when transgender activists in Malaysia were publicly seeking legal rights to be interpreted as allowing those who were transgender or third gender to formally change their identification. This was articulated by someone from the PLHIV/NGO community in that transgender people are supported when it comes to HIV prevention but not within the legal domain of human rights and recognition of their identity:

For their health not for their rights. That is different. For their health, for their HIV prevention, yes we support them [transgender people].But asking for their right and these things. I cannot agree with that. (14, PLHIV)

There is a quandary posed by raising the issue of human rights as it highlights a crucially important distinction in some people's minds: that health trumps human rights. In addition, it signifies that perhaps there are some areas of HIV prevention policy that certain stakeholders are not comfortable with but are nevertheless required to adhere to so as to tow the party line. Some participants from within the Ministry of Health had the view that human rights were not fixed but debatable and that human rights must have some boundaries:

I try to say, right of a person not to be infected. People came talking about human rights issues and their perspective of human right. The other perspective of human rights must be effected. The human rights must have a boundary. (3, Ministry of Health)

The excerpt elucidates how the argument of denial of human rights is quashed, by arguing that other rights reign supreme and that the right to prevent someone being infected with HIV justifies certain policies designed to prevent HIV, for example pre-marital HIV screening.

There was also recognition among some interviewees that there were other rights within Malaysia which were seen as lacking, such as the rights of women, because of patriarchy and polygamy, and that these factors also needed to be addressed:

It's a man's world. (16, PLHIV)

Furthermore, there was cognisance by some participants that although LGBT rights needed to be recognised, such issues have now become inextricably linked with politics and religion, tainting the actual discussion and making it much more polemic and sensational than is necessary:

Challenges are many; I mean you look at today the whole issue LGBT which has been politicised, you know, by religious people, by politicians actually, you need to recognise the existence of LGBT. (16, PLHIV)

Differing viewpoints on issues such as human rights are some of the factors, amongst many, which have strained stakeholder relationships.

Stakeholder Relationships

There were obvious and more subtle strains and tensions between the various stakeholders and even within those from the same stakeholder group. Questions arose from the interviews that spark discussions surrounding which stakeholder possessed the most power and influence, who were the actual policy makers and perceptions of stakeholders.

The Ministry of Health was seen as the main policy maker in HIV prevention as a governmental agency and having the most power and influence. Those participants interviewed from within the Ministry of Health expressed a sense of being under pressure arising from having to be accountable, to serve and be mindful of the PLHIV/NGO and at risk community:

Not only the marginalised community but the people at large, because we are using their budget. We are getting the budget with the tax payers' money, so we are answerable. (10, Ministry of Health)

Not only is the Ministry of Health accountable to the government and tax paying Malaysian citizens but they also have to be aware that, for the most part, the health care providers who, for example, may distribute condoms are Muslim and are subject to their own opinions which may, or may not, influence health care provision:

It's not easy because you know that the health care providers, majority are Muslims. (10, Ministry of Health)

Hence, the Ministry of Health felt it had to be realistic and mindful when creating strategies of who will be implementing their policies. Participants from the Ministry of Health felt that they had to reconcile their dual role of a public health physician with their personal role of being a Muslim and these roles were felt to be in conflict when issues such as condom use came into discussion:

OK, I'm a Muslim, I am a doctor. (25, Ministry of Health)

Therefore, the Ministry of Health had to negotiate and reinterpret its actions to itself and also to its colleagues. The best strategy to circumvent this was by not asking too many questions as to whether those receiving condoms were married, heterosexual or homosexual, thus obviating the onus of responsibility:

We are rather quiet about the behaviour but personally, I can say that as long as we are Muslim, we don't agree with the behaviour. But we are trying to be professional in our work here, we are looking at the transmission part, we are wearing different hats. (10, Ministry of Health)

Those working in the Ministry of Health all had their own personal views about condoms and sexual acts that they thought were sinful but had to balance their religious objections with their professional capacity. Some of those participants also felt that they were culpable in that sin too (by distributing condoms etc), a concept of *shubhah*. As Muslims, they felt that they had a religious obligation to condemn the acts which contravene the teachings of Islam, such as *zina*, but could not do so outwardly because of their professional role. This meant they had to repress their own disquiet on the matter and effectively outsource the religious duty to groups such as JAKIM:

We are not touching on the issues on the sinful acts, rather the transmission part, we leave that, that's why we work hand in hand with JAKIM because it is their duty to tackle on the other part. (10, Ministry of Health)

The response to the Ministry of Health shown by other stakeholders ranged from silence to subtle mocking, and members of the Ministry were often aware of the perception other stakeholder groups had about them:

So the views which I get is that we are not doing enough. (25, Ministry of Health)

It was clear that those with higher leadership roles within the PLHIV and those who represented PLHIV had strained relationships with the Ministry of Health. PLHIV deemed themselves as having little bargaining power in terms of influencing policy. The Malaysian Aids Council (MAC) is widely considered to be the umbrella organisation which represents the various HIV NGOs but almost half of its funding is obtained through the Ministry of Health. This was in contrast to other participants who had not been granted funding for work with high risk groups, such as MSM:

The government doesn't give funding, especially like, for example, in our community for MSM; they don't tend to give funding to us. (19, PLHIV)

Such actions heavily influenced relationships with stakeholders and government, creating an environment where civil society cannot really speak up as there are ramifications and consequences for doing so.

Amongst the PLHIV group, religious leaders were seen as unhelpful in their HIV prevention activities and their promotion of abstinence of sexual activity and cessation of drug use was seen as over simplistic:

> Not too helpful in the way to prevent HIV, they [religious leaders] just can say this, OK, stop doing sexual activity, OK it's time for you to stop, stop being a drug user. (22, PLHIV)

> When I talk to the imams they say OK, why you giving condoms, why you giving, why we can't go via the spiritual ways of managing this? But for me, we are looking at what's the best practices in the context of public health. (15, PLHIV)

For the most part, religious leaders did not agree with the PLHIV prevention activities. Furthermore, those at the coalface felt uncomfortable speaking with *ustads* (religious leaders) because of a sense of shame (*malu*), either perceived or real. Negative experiences of other PLHIV interacting with religious leaders often reverberated in the community so that even if the person in question did not have a first-hand unpleasant experience of religious leaders, their perception of religious leaders was irreversibly influenced. The so called 'conversion' *muhayam* camps had damaged relations between PLHIV and religious leaders. However, from the margins of the PLHIV community, highly atypically, it was felt that they themselves had not had reached out effectively to the religious leaders and the Ministry of Health:

> We fail also to understand where these people [religious leaders and MOH] are coming from; what are we doing to convince them? (16, PLHIV)

The above quote is important as it recognises that the other stakeholders have their own interests and agendas and that one must engage with them.

> I mean, this country is always like that, from top down. Government works in silos. (23, PLHIV)

The top down approach was considered the norm; however, there was one atypical viewpoint from someone who believed that power was bottom up because citizens can raise issues in parliament:

> Malaysia is a democracy country and it's bottom up. (15, PLHIV)

The PLHIV community represents a minority; any possible influence in parliament is limited by the mathematics of numerical representation. This bottom up approach can work against PLHIV when the majority Malay Muslim population disagrees with certain HIV prevention approaches and raises the issue in parliament. PLHIV's perception of their own power and influence was low and subjugated to a high degree as PLHIV felt their viewpoint was not heard and was considered irrelevant in discussions with government, whereas outside forces such as the UN were listened to:

> As an NGO, if you were to tell the Government, the Government wouldn't event look at you, wouldn't even listen to you, but for example you have UN agencies doing it, they take a different view of it, you know, they will listen. (16, PLHIV)

Religious leaders were aware that they had an important role to play in terms of education and awareness of HIV but their stance on prevention was to promote Islamic values to tackle HIV:

We from JAKIM part that the main programme is about awareness. We go on ground to the peoples, meet peoples like being out of reach and then give them the awareness programme. It's not things that sounds like the Ministry of Health has done. They give the condom. (2, Religious Leader)

This was a defining feature for many religious leaders and it was clear that they did not agree with the stance of the Ministry of Health with regards to the distribution of condoms; however, they did not stand in its way. Their modus operandi was significantly different in approach to prevention of HIV and was consistent with their own values and views of the responsibility of JAKIM and imams to explain and propagate Islam:

We must go back to Islam, go back to *ibaadat* (prayer). (33, Religious Leader)

However, some religious leaders, an atypical view albeit, were concerned at how they were perceived by PLHIV and worried that Islam itself or religious bodies would be deemed too strict and could possibly push those away from Islam:

The people living with HIV or LGBT group don't judge Islam, Islamic body or Islamic Department. (17, Religious Leader)

This participant was aware that there were tensions between religious leaders and PLHIV and was aware that the *muhayam* camp programme was seen as a cause of conflict, distrust and tension between the two stakeholders:

PT officer tell *muhayyam* is to transform and I say 'no'; *muhayyam* the meaning is camping. (17, Religious Leader)

Although some participants felt that religious leaders were obstructing HIV interventions, some stakeholders were sympathetic to their position:

People thought also in those years that sometime religions can be the hindering factors for HIV interventions. So it's not so. People perceive that but it's not so. (3, Ministry of Health)

With regards to which stakeholders influence policy making, the perception was that the Ministry of Health had the greatest influence; this was a typical response.

Ministry of Health, I think, the Education Ministry also. (14, PLHIV)

Other stakeholders were deemed to include governmental ministries such as the Ministry of Education and the Ministry of Religion. An atypical response stipulated not just the governmental religious bodies, such as JAKIM, but also the head of the state, the Sultan. The Ministry of Education was often mentioned by the Ministry of Health as being completely responsible for sex education, which was therefore considered outside of the remit of the Ministry of Health. However, some perceived that the Ministry of Education was pandering to popular opinion:

The Ministry of Education only always thinks about what other people think but it's not about the logic about it. (19, PLHIV)

An atypical response from the Ministry of Health was that the situation was far more complicated than just their input but included local government and the housing ministry as well as the police. There were also a number of unprompted discussions among the participants about who should be ultimately responsible for HIV prevention. There was a general consensus from the Ministry of Health that the issue of preventing HIV was a mandate that could not feasibly be fulfilled by the Ministry of Health alone and that the responsibility should ultimately be widened to everyone. This included not only governmental departments, such as the Department of Religion, but also religious organisations, communities and civil societies including the NGO sector:

> Putting HIV as the responsibility of everyone because there is no one organisation or Ministry or body can really control and prevent the spread. (31, Ministry of Health)

There was a sense within the Ministry of Health that there were unreasonable expectations being placed on them to interfere in issues which were not within their remit, such as laws:

> You can't ask me to change the law. I can't do it; I have not been in the parliament. I can't, I can't do much. (3, Ministry of Health)

> HIV is not just, it's not just Ministry of Health's responsibility; it comes also under the Ministry of Education, social welfare and so and so. (25, Ministry of Health)

Sex education was another example with each sector deeming the other should take on a more concrete role, with no one holding responsibility, in the belief that a multi-sector approach is required. However, in order for such a multi-sector approach to be achievable, each sector needs to be able to work together in a coordinated way, yet there was appreciation that different stakeholders worked in isolation and not in partnership.

Actions to be Taken by Stakeholders

The perception amongst the Ministry of Health was that their strategy thus far had been reasonably good in preventing cases of HIV and they felt continuing in the same trajectory was fair:

> Majority of our strategy – I think we are on the right path OK. (25, Ministry of Health)

However, the other stakeholders felt there was much more that could be done and recommendations and advice ranged from concrete suggestions to more abstract ideas or a shift in attitudes. Importantly, all stakeholders expressed a genuine interest and commitment to preventing HIV in Malaysia; however, unsurprisingly, they all had very different action plans on how that objective could be achieved.

There was a prevalent opinion amongst the religious leaders that the current HIV prevention policies did not address the root cause of the problem but rather just alleviated the signs and symptoms by needle exchange or condom distribution. The majority of the religious leaders felt that HIV was a symptom of wider issues in society that could be eliminated, or at least reduced, by following the teachings and rules of Islam, which prohibit sex outside marriage:

This is number one. Pray, follow Islam rule. (34, Religious Leader)

The insistence to 'pray' and follow the rules of Islam relate to HIV prevention specifically and not HIV treatment. No conflict was seen between taking antiretroviral medication to treat HIV and praying to *Allah* for good health. This is important to note because in some other religious contexts outside of Malaysia there have been those who felt that true faith meant not using Western medicines and solely praying.

There were differing opinions regarding whether there was a need for relationship or sex education in the first place, and, if there was, what type, where and who should be responsible for its implementation. Across all stakeholders there was the view that greater effort needed to be made in educating people about HIV. Some participants believed this should be a community effort and should be initiated from a younger age in schools:

I think everybody should to be involved. NGO, the Government, the Ministry of Health, everybody, in schools, they should start the sex education. (22, PLHIV MSM)

Some participants deemed that the onus of responsibility was on the Ministry of Education to provide sex education programmes within schools:

Ministry of Education should give sex education in high school. Starting from high school, because that's when people know about this. (19, PLHIV)

Other participants, such as the Ministry of Health, accepted that there needed to be some sort of health education in schools as well as in universities, but did not specifically call it 'sex education':

About HIV, education starts at school; clubs and schools, you know, which are aimed to advise them on high risk sexual behaviour. (11, Ministry of Health)

However, it was not clarified who would implement or be responsible for such a programme which was rather a somewhat vague wish. Other participants, such as religious leaders, were clearer and simply felt that specific and correct information about how HIV was transmitted was important:

You have to convey correct information. (9, Religious Leader)

For many of the participants from the PLHIV community, the way forward was to use condoms to prevent HIV, either by increasing their access and information about them or by assisting those who provide these, such as NGOs:

When you have sex, you should use condom. (4, PLHIV Transgender Woman)

Many of the transgender participants were keen to promote condom usage for themselves and for others.

I mean to avoid people getting HIV, condom. (5, PLHIV Transgender Woman)

Some within the PLHIV community felt that the Ministry of Health distribution of condom scheme was haphazard, as although it did provide condoms it was no longer providing lubricants which for those in the MSM community who practise anal sex was hugely important:

> They do provide condoms but unfortunately this year they, Ministry of Health cut the funding for lubricant; they only provide condom, because I heard that they say that they don't want to make the session become more enjoyable … So these two should be together, condom and lubricant. (22, PLHIV MSM)

Many of the participants felt that adequate measures needed to be taken to curb the stigma and discrimination faced by those living with HIV and the perception of HIV by society:

> No more stigma and discrimination … our people outside there can accept me because they don't know I am a PLHIV. If they know I am a PLHIV, I think they don't want to share a plate with me. (26, PLHIV)

For PLHIV as people who habitually experience the ramifications of stigma, tackling this issue was seen as a key priority area. Furthermore, the stigma and discrimination was seen to be at an institutional level by the police and enforcement agency. Such actions were seen as creating a hostile environment where HIV prevention activities were more difficult to implement.

Some participants were resolute that if you change the laws first, HIV prevention on the ground would be easier to facilitate:

> We have far too many policies and laws – dealing with drug users, sex workers and MSM – that are not supportive of good HIV prevention programs at a large scale. (32, PLHIV)

This was a typical view from those within the PLHIV community stakeholder group, namely that an enabling environment needed to be facilitated. However, it is important to note that some participants from other stakeholder groups vehemently disagreed with that stance and felt that issues of law and discrimination by police had been blown out of proportion by the PLHIV community and that human rights groups and the 'police were doing their job' (25, Ministry of Health). This is central to why those from the PLHIV community argue that laws need to change, because the police may indeed only be 'doing their job', and enforcement of those laws hampers HIV prevention programmes.

There was a high level of mutual trust from those within the PLHIV community who are also service users of the various NGOs. Their work was seen as crucial for HIV prevention and a sense prevailed that the NGOs could reach the areas that other organisations could not. Thus, providing support to these organisations to continue their services was really vital to HIV prevention. Whether this support was in financial terms or in some other form was not clearly articulated by participants, but it was emphasised that the government must support the NGOs:

> Our government must give 100 percent support to all NGO. (6, PLHIV Transgender Woman)

Some participants felt that those living with HIV needed to be re-humanised in Malaysian society:

> OK, I just want to say we are PLHIV, we are person too. (26, PLHIV)

HIV was seen by some as something that happened only to 'other' people, not to family, friends or people whom you would meet on a regular basis. Such thinking essentially dehumanised those with HIV and that climate indirectly affected HIV prevention in Malaysia. The media were often seen as a factor which influenced the negative portrayal of people with HIV in society:

> And again, I think the media does not help that much. Because the portrayal of HIV I think is always negative, the other problem I feel that needs to be corrected in Malaysia is, we should not be judgemental. This is based on my own perception. I see that people tend to judge those with HIV. (1, Religious Leader)

Some participants had the belief that HIV was simply not on the radar of the average Malaysian with people simply not considering HIV was still a pressing problem:

> Public education campaigns that reminds people it's [HIV] still here. (23, PLHIV)

It was seen as crucial by those in the PLHIV community to actively increase awareness of HIV amongst the general public so that the myths surrounding HIV transmission, such as the notion that HIV could be passed on from sharing a plate of food, could be dispelled. In addition, it was felt that the actual methods of transmission of HIV could be explained to society not only for prevention and education purposes but also to mitigate stigma and discrimination. Other participants felt that as part of awareness and education, there should be encouragement for sex workers to actively seek testing for HIV. This collegiality suggests that peer education, already practised by some NGOs, would be highly valuable:

> You have to have a programme, workshop on prevention, how HIV transmits, the transmission, prevention, and also she, as an old person, she would advise all her friends who do sex working to go for test, go for test to make sure that you are safe, don't be shy. (6, PLHIV Transgender Woman)

It was mentioned by those living with HIV that religious leaders could be utilised and galvanised to educate the Malaysian Muslim communities about HIV and AIDS in religious sermons:

> In the Friday prayers they should talk jn *khutbah* how to prevent HIV and AIDS, they do talk about HIV and AIDS but it's only a once a year. (22, PLHIV)

Religious leaders were seen as particularly useful in more rural areas which were often hard to reach, where they had greater access to local populations and were highly revered by members of the community.

One of the key features mentioned by participants across the stakeholders was an attitudinal shift:

> I think, number one, everyone should not be in denial. I think that's the most important step that should be taken. Once we deny that there is a problem, then we will stop looking for solutions. (1, Religious Leader)

There was a perception that this sense of denial needed to be replaced with an environment of openness in a culturally and religiously sensitive manner and this was particularly the case with regard to sex and relationships education in schools:

> Sex education at school, in my time, not much sex education in school. Malay culture, they are not too open about sex, but for me when we talk about HIV, we must talk about sex. (6, PLHIV Transgender Woman)

However, some religious leaders took a diametrically opposite view that Malaysian society should be less open, as talking about such issues like premarital sex and transgender women would lead to more cases of HIV:

> Must not be open, there will be more TGs. (33, Religious Leader)

This response, although atypical, is still significant as it shows the mentality which exists amongst some stakeholders:

> A question of religious attitudes, mentality that comes at every step of the campaign, the question of religious taboos and mentality. (9, Religious Leader)

There was also a culture amongst the stakeholders of blaming the Ministry of Health, and one another, and this was felt to be counterproductive and simply wasted time. One participant from the Ministry of Health demanded 'don't blame' (25, Ministry of Health).

Casting blame was seen as damaging already fragile stakeholder relationships and networks which were constantly fractious under the surface. Other participants from the PLHIV community interestingly felt it was essential for the Ministry of Health and the leadership therein to be more professional and target those most at risk:

> The Ministry of Health needs to adopt a more scientific public health approach when it comes to implementing their programs and prioritise. (32, PLHIV)

Other Themes

There were a number of overarching themes in the interviews, such as language, comparison of the East with the West and the rural and urban divide as well as the perception of the patient who is innocent. In combination they give support to the value of an anthropological understanding of the situation in Malaysia, illustrating that no health issues, certainly not ones to do with HIV, exist without a complex underplay of politics and historical antecedents.

The terms and expressions used during the interviews were particularly illuminating in understanding the perceptions of stakeholders that were not overtly expressed. Language was used as a way of negotiation and damage limitation as well as being diplomatic and helping appease stakeholders. For example, expressions such as 'human rights' were seen as a polemical term, as a Western idea with negative connotations. As a corollary to this, human rights groups were seen often by some participants as a nuisance and interfering. Furthermore, human rights in the

Western sense of the term was often seen by religious leaders as incompatible with Islam, which had historically had its own comprehensive system of ensuring justice and 'rights'.

'Free sex' was a term used to describe the sexual patterns and norm of the West, which was depicted by religious leaders as sexually frenetic, casual and hence promoted a fear that being 'open' to sex education would lead to the moral degeneration of core Malaysian Islamic values. Sometimes, the language used was confusing, even contradictory, such as with regards to the policy of pre-marital HIV testing where the word 'mandatory' was interchanged by certain interviewees with 'voluntary'. Some language was intentionally employed to be more diplomatic and acceptable. However, there was much usage of words such as 'prostitution' and 'sodomy' by religious leaders and, at times, by Ministry of Health officials working in the HIV/AIDS department. For many, 'prostitution' implies judgement and has long been replaced by the term 'sex work'. Sodomy is also considered an anachronistic word and is seldom used by those in the HIV field; instead, 'anal sex' is used.

There was awareness among some that the use of terms such as 'prostitution', especially by those in the Ministry of Health, who were Muslim but should appear to be neutral, impartial and non-judgemental, was incorrect. Indeed, there were occasions where participants self-corrected their terminology:

> … because prostitution as such, I mean professional sex workers. (11, Ministry of Health)

Using alternate language may be a bridge to negotiating reconciliation and stakeholder collaboration or at least using a standard language referencing code. Also noticeable was the language that was used to define groups, such as the abbreviation 'PLU' (People Like Us) used by the MSM community.

> … we call it as PLU, means 'people like us'. (19, PLHIV MSM)

This implied an 'us' and 'them' mentality, seen also with transgender women, and highlights the pervasive divisions within the subgroups of the population. Some of the language used to describe PLHIV could be perceived as judgemental, the term 'innocent victims (11, Ministry of Health), for example. This implies a dichotomy between those who are 'innocent victims' and acquire HIV through legal means and those who are perceived to be deserving of blame and have HIV as a consequence of sinful or illegal actions, such as sex work for instance:

> I declare my status and my head of religious can accept me and give a support to me and my family. They know I get from my late husband because my late husband passed away with AIDS symptoms. (27, PLHIV Housewife)

The lady described above had a rather more positive experience than many PLHIV but acknowledges that this was most likely because the community was aware she was infected by her husband, and was therefore not blameworthy. This also has ramifications for funding; those who are seen as 'innocent victims' are perhaps easier to market for funding as opposed to the high risk groups of MSM, transgender individuals and sex workers, who are seen as culpable but yet where the greatest need exists. There was also from some a reframing of HIV prevention activities, such as condom distribution, under disease prevention and a more biomedical, scientific way of interpretation:

> Disease prevention, as under disease prevention, so we don't go into the moral aspects of it as health workers. (11, Ministry of Health)

Condom distribution is one of the most controversial policies to prevent HIV in Malaysia and is not approved of by religious leaders; thus, redefining the issue as a response to a health problem, a mechanism of disease prevention, rather than looking at it as a moral issue appeases various factions. Such diplomacy reasserts that preventing HIV is a public health issue not a social one when in interaction with stakeholders, as preservation of health is considered as a central value throughout the history of science and medicine in the Islamic world.

More generally, there was often reference to the West in comparison to Malaysia, the East, from the various stakeholders; the West was often looked upon negatively, seen as morally degenerate in terms of sexual behaviour and 'free sex', the antithesis of what the country of Malaysia aspired to be; hence, the fear of 'safe sex' education messages in schools proliferated. On the other hand, the West was seen by those within the PLHIV community positively, as an idyll of diversity and inclusion:

> How are people like us treated there, in the outside world? That's why I sometimes I say, why still people degrade us. In overseas wow! You know Andrej Pejic? The one very famous model. (5, PLHIV Transgender Woman)

Finally, this study was undertaken looking at an urban area, though some of the people interviewed may not have always been a resident there and some have experience or grew up in a more rural surrounding, in the village 'Kampung':

> Yes, when we stay in our village, in Kampung, our resident there cannot accept when we have HIV positive. Discrimination in Malaysia culture, in Islam they are not too open about this disease, except when except when we live in a town; in a village we see this issue is not too open. (26, PLHIV MSM)

Quantitative Results

Demography of Respondents

There were 252 participants in the quantitative component of the study, completing the self-administered questionnaire, with three stakeholder groups: religious leaders, people living with HIV and the Ministry of Health, abbreviated as RL, PLHIV and MOH respectively. The largest group of participants comprised PLHIV, followed by religious leaders and then the Ministry of Health with 28 participants (Table 4.1).

Participants had a median age of 34; 51.0% identified themselves as males, 42.9% as female, and 6.1% as transgender. 9.0% achieved attained primary education only, 41.5% up to secondary and 49.6% up to tertiary level. The Ministry of Health had a greater proportion of education up to tertiary level (75%), religious

Table 4.1 Distribution of stakeholder group surveyed

Stakeholder	Number	Percent
MOH	28	11
PLHIV	117	46
RL	107	43
Total	252	100

leaders (49.5%) compared to the PLHIV group which was (35.9%) and this difference in distribution in educational level across the three stakeholder groups is statistically significant using chi-squared testing (p < 0.001).

Correct Knowledge of HIV Transmission

In the questionnaire, respondents were asked how HIV could be transmitted. These answers were scored for correctness, either 0 (incorrect) or 1 (correct). The highest possible score was 14 and lowest was 0. The scores obtained across respondents ranged from 1 to 14, with mean and median scores of 11 and 12 respectively. Bivariate analysis was undertaken to look at the scores across subgroups, such as stakeholder or level or education, and findings were tested for significance using non-parametric tests.

When analysed, according to stakeholder group, the Ministry of Health scored highest, then PLHIV and finally religious leaders (Table 4.2). Significance testing was conducted using the Kruskall-Wallis test (p < 0.001) and it was found that there was a statistically significant difference between the knowledge scores of HIV transmission across the three stakeholder groups.

When knowledge scores of HIV transmission were analysed according to education level, there was a difference with those respondents who achieved tertiary level education scoring highest, then secondary and then primary (medians 12, 11 and 11 respectively and means 11.9, 10.8 and 10.7 respectively). This was statistically significant when testing using the Kruskal-Wallis test (p = 0.001).

The distribution of knowledge of HIV transmission differed across the genders with males scoring highest, followed by females followed by 'other' (transgender women) (medians 12, 12 and 11 respectively and means 11.6, 11.1 and 9.9 respectively). This was statistically significant using the Kruskal-Wallis test (p = 0.004).

There was no significant difference in scores across age groups.

When all variables were controlled for in a multiple linear regression, it was found that only higher education was associated with a higher knowledge of HIV scores (p = 0.014).

Table 4.2 Correct knowledge of HIV transmission across stakeholder groups

Stakeholder group	Correct knowledge score mean	Correct knowledge score median
MOH	12.7	13
PLHIV	11.3	12
RL	10.9	11

Correct Knowledge of HIV Prevention

In the questionnaire, respondents were asked about possible measures which could prevent HIV infection. Their answers were scored for correctness and aggregated, giving a composite score for each respondent, with the lowest score possible being 0 and the highest being 6. The scores obtained indeed ranged from 0 to 6 with a mean of 4.8 and a median of 5.

There was a difference in distribution of knowledge across the Ministry of Health, religious leaders and PLHIV. Those from the Ministry of Health scored highest, followed by religious leaders and then PLHIV (medians 6, 5 and 5 respectively and means 5.7, 4.7 and 4.7 respectively). This was statistically significant using the Kruskal-Wallis test (p = 0.001).

There were no statistically significant differences in HIV knowledge prevention scores with respect to age or gender.

HIV prevention knowledge scores of respondents differed across education levels; those educated up to tertiary level scored highest, followed by secondary and then primary (medians 5, 5 and 5 respectively and means 5.03, 4.6 and 4.6). This difference was found to be statistically significant using the Kruskal-Wallis test (p = 0.004).

After all variables were controlled for by performing a multiple linear regression, only higher education was found to be associated with higher knowledge of HIV prevention scores (p = 0.023).

When the composite knowledge scores for both HIV transmission and prevention were broken down by individual questions, there were some noteworthy findings as revealed using chi-squared analysis.

There was a statistically significant difference (p < 0.001) across stakeholders in the proportions that correctly answered whether HIV could be transmitted through insect bites, with Ministry of Health scoring highest at 93%, followed by PLHIV at 87% and religious leaders at 59%.

There was a statistically significant difference in the proportion who correctly answered the question relating to whether HIV can be prevented through condom usage during sexual activity. PLHIV scored highest at 92%, followed by Ministry of Health at 89% and religious leaders at 77% (p = 0.007).

Sources of HIV Knowledge

Finally, the varying sources of information whereby people stated that they had obtained information regarding HIV can be ranked:

1. HIV information from web   (73%)
2. HIV information from MOH   (72%)
3. HIV information from TV   (69%)
4. HIV information from newspaper   (62%)
5. HIV information from healthcare worker   (56%)
6. HIV information from radio   (44%)
7. HIV information from other printed   (30%)
8. HIV information from billboard   (29%)

It is clear that the three most common sources of information amongst the respondents arose from the internet, the Ministry of Health and TV.

Chapter 5
Discussion

Context

Malaysia is one of the countries in South East Asia with a primarily Muslim majority population, where people practise their faith in Islam openly as well as privately, consistent with local culture. However, there are many Muslims worldwide and they are not a homogenous group but are highly heterogonous, differing in terms of culture, belief and practice of Islam. Sheikh Lemu of the Islamic Education Trust (2015) explains succinctly that though 'there exists a diversity of opinion amongst Muslim scholars' but that these 'differences do not imply disunity'. People practise Islam, as well as interpret Islam in various ways across the world, clearly pointed out by one of the religious leaders interviewed:

> Islam as a religion and local customs has to be mixed; you cannot get rid of that. (24, Religious Leader)

Even within Malaysia, widely acknowledged to be on the whole quite observant to Islam, there exists differing degrees and manifestations of Islamic practice and a myriad of so called 'Islamic viewpoints' from religious leaders, ranging from the orthodox conservative, through moderate, to the more progressive and liberal. For those who do practise Islam to a greater or lesser degree, Islam is not seen in a compartmentalized way, as in a secular country, but as incorporating not just religious duties to be undertaken in private or in the company of a minority of others but also actions in the public sphere. Islam was seen as all encompassing, regarding 'body' and 'soul', as described by one of the religious leaders interviewed:

> The health of the human being was not divided into the health of his body full stop. But, it was both the health of his body as well as the health of his soul. (35, Religious Leader)

In the views of the interviewees, Islam extended to being interested in the health of the community, society, *ummah* and mankind. Furthermore, the role of Islam was

© The Author(s) 2018
S. Barmania, M.J. Reiss, *Islam and Health Policies Related
to HIV Prevention in Malaysia*, SpringerBriefs in Public Health,
https://doi.org/10.1007/978-3-319-68909-8_5

privy to private matters of conjugal rights and intimate sexual activities and behaviour, with Islamic teachings pertaining to premarital and extra-marital sex.

Islamic Religious Belief and Sexual Behaviour

To fully understand the influence of Islamic religious beliefs on sexual behaviour and HIV policy one must first understand its influence at a macroscopic level.

Islam is seen as a way of life, which encompasses both private and public domain. Importance is placed on the intention (*niyat*) of an individual to submit to God's will and worship him. Furthermore, worshiping God in Islam includes following the comprehensive set of rules, regulations and commands on both how to pray and also how to conduct yourself in daily life as set forth in the *Qur'an* and *Sunnah*. There are rules with regards to eating, fasting, charity and cleanliness as well as those relating to sexual behaviour, with some activities forbidden (*haram*) whilst others are allowed (*halal*). During the course of the interviews, there was a clear sentiment that the rules were there to protect the individual from harm for their own benefit ('life and intellect'). Also, there was an understanding expressed by participants, mostly by the religious leaders, that the rules were there to protect the community in the future, to prevent social ills, simplify issues such as lineage, to strengthen and safeguard the Muslim *ummah* and above all to prevent harm. This is articulated by the excerpt below by an official from the Ministry of Health:

> The whole Quran is a way of preventing harm in a wider sense, whether to body or society as a whole. (25, Ministry of Health)

In Islam, sex outside the confines and sanctity of marriage is wholly forbidden; sexual activity has to be governed, guiding Muslims as to which are and are not acceptable sexual practices. In particular, engaging in sexual activity for financial remuneration, as in sex work, is forbidden. In Malaysia, Islam is a matter for the state as well as under the purview of *Sharia* law and some sexual activities such as those considered in Section 377 are in the penal code (UN 2014); this means that they are thus not simply morally or religiously forbidden but also considered criminal.

Sex before marriage (*zina*) was forbidden; those who wished to engage in such activity were simply encouraged to get married. However, Malaysia was not seen as a society which was strictly segregated by gender as is the case in other Muslim countries; men and women are educated in schools and universities together, as well as working professionally and there were opportunities for sexual activity to occur. The reality is that people, for whatever reason, did not always behave in terms of sexual activity as they were supposed to, even if they were Muslim. The ideal of how Muslims should behave according to Islam is not always in keeping with reality. During the interviews with the stakeholders it was apparent that there were a number of ways that people in Malaysian society responded to those who acted out of the normal sexual boundaries, exemplified by the excerpt below:

> But because of the misconception and looking into HIV as a sin, it's a product of sinful action right? That's why the magnitude of stigma and discrimination is really very huge in Malaysia. (31, Ministry of Health)

One approach was to demonise and chastise, either publicly or in private, those who acted against the rules of Islam with HIV seen as a product of sinful behaviour, a punishment. This contributes to the stigma and discrimination experienced by those with HIV. For those who are undertaking sexual activity which is not in line with Islam, it meant that there was a sense of shame (*malu*) and they were more likely to go underground, especially for those Men who are have Sex with Men, who are often also married to a woman.

Many interviewed participants said that Malaysian and Islamic society was less open about sex outside marriage and that talking about such things was taboo and akin to encouraging it. Some of the religious leaders were keen to explain that there is a strong idea in Islam that one must not expose the failings or sins of others as this is between the individual and the Creator. However, what may originate as an honourable wish to 'cover the sin' can lead rather innocuously to a climate of silence and denial.

As it was not anticipated or expected by society that a young Malaysian would engage in premarital sex or homosexuality it seemed unnecessary to offer any sex education apart from that which was provided on the premarital counselling course. However, there were some cases in the study which showed that those young adults who had engaged in sex were ill-prepared and had little information.

It is important to note that beliefs about Islam are interpreted and explained by religious leaders, *imams* and *ustads* in Malaysia. There are different religious viewpoints, a spectrum that exists along the line of liberal to strict and this was evident amongst the religious leaders who were interviewed as a core stakeholder group. There were leaders who showed a more progressive viewpoint through to those who were more staunch and conservative. These attitudes manifested themselves in relation to discussions on Islamic religious beliefs pertaining to sexual behaviour and HIV prevention. It was not in dispute that sex outside marriage was forbidden; this belief was commonplace; however, there was a spectrum of views amongst the Islamic religious leaders who participated as to what was the correct way of dealing with such situations. This often correlated with education levels, with those more academic in nature being more progressive but this was not always the case as there were certainly exceptions to that pattern.

In fact, one religious leader, academic and highly educated, was particularly conservative, admitting that if a person followed the rules HIV simply would not occur and that 'someone who commits *zina* should be killed'. However, even amongst those religious leaders who were very conservative, there was still a genuine wish not to want those affected with HIV to dissociate from the 'Islamic community'.

One religious leader seemed highly reluctant to perform burial procedures (*janaza*) on those who died due to the consequence of AIDS. Interestingly, there are some religious organisations, such as JAKIM, that actively teach and train religious leaders on how to bury those with HIV (no different from a usual Muslim burial), and this highlights some of the important work that religious leaders do in connection with HIV, providing services where other religious leaders shy away.

Some religious leaders felt that there is an element of choice in Islam, personal free will to choose to make the right decisions in accordance with the teachings of Islam and this pertains to issues of sexual activity and behaviour. Such leaders felt there should be some distance between the state and religious practice and that it was not the remit of the state to mandate for such personal issues. However, such a viewpoint tended to be held by a minority who ultimately believed that Islam was not solely following rules, but understanding the intentions and principles behind them.

Such leaders were keen to propagate the sentiment that Islam was a very practical religion and that there had been a great debate about the revival of some principles mentioned in Islam such as that of *maslaha* (issues of public interest), the idea of the greater and lesser of two harms (*darar*) and *isthihad* (independent decision making).

In the context of HIV in Malaysia, a large majority of those infected arise from Men who have Sex with Men, transgender communities and sex workers, actions and behaviours that are emphatically at odds and forbidden in Islam (Obermeyer 2006). How does a country and policy makers create a strategy that is in keeping with Islamic religious beliefs about sexual behaviour as well as adequately ensure that HIV is prevented from spreading? The influence of Islam is hugely significant, ubiquitous and encompasses all those who are working in the field—those who make the policies as well as those who are recipients of the services, Non-Governmental Organisations, religious leaders and the Ministry of Health.

The significance of Islam on HIV prevention policy is directly related to the different mechanisms proposed and advocated by the different stakeholders as each has its own distinctive view on how HIV can and should be prevented. For example, the stakeholders from the religious group fundamentally believe that the only long-term way of reducing the prevalence of HIV is by 'going back to Islam', an expression heard frequently during the interviews. This includes the promotion of abstinence from sexual activity until marriage and most certainly does not condone or endorse safer sexual practices outside of marriage, such as condom distribution, as this contradicts their central belief system.

Within the Ministry of Health, a different viewpoint is taken that endeavours to be more public health focussed, in favour of the distribution of condoms. However, it must be noted that individuals within the Ministry of Health themselves have their own Islamic perspectives and are subject to questioning by other groups, including religious leaders and individual tax paying Malaysian Muslim citizens.

Furthermore, Islam affects not just health policy and power but also the process and the manner in which policies are implemented and this is apparent in the way in which the premarital HIV screening test came to existence, namely that it is necessary for Muslim married couples but not non-Muslims. There are certain tactics utilized to simply and crudely 'get things done', as expressed by a number of participants. This either meant that activities of certain programmes, such as HIV prevention ones within the NGO community that were targeted at marginal groups, for example, Men who have Sex with Men, had either to be done 'silently' or at least not in a way that overtly advertised their work, otherwise such activities can jeopardise other stake-holders and even funding.

In such cases, it was noticeable how important language is and how it was used to neutralise and placate stakeholders, by focussing on health rather than rights, with adoption of the term favoured by the Ministry of Health, namely, 'prevention of disease'.

Furthermore, although Malaysia's predominant population consists of Muslims, many who are living with HIV or are at risk of HIV infection are not; yet, they also are influenced by Islamic religious beliefs on HIV prevention policies and one can ask whether their needs are met. However, perhaps this discrepancy could be seen as an asset and a way of circumventing the rules, by reiterating the statement that it is not just Muslims who are affected by HIV but non-Muslims too, and that as Malaysia is a multicultural, multi-ethnic and multi-religious society, the government and health policies must be suitable for them too.

This raises the question of who are the stakeholders who are instrumental in designing these HIV prevention policies and who have the most influence and power? There is a certain body of thought that holds that whoever has the greatest influence certainly does not include those PLHIV themselves, as is indicated in this study.

Power Dynamics

There is a definite schism in the balance of power between PLHIV group, and those who are supposed to represent them, and other stakeholders, mainly religious leaders and the Ministry of Health, both groups of which come under the jurisdiction of the government. During the course of the interviews, there was a strong sense and acknowledgement that Malaysia worked in a very hierarchal fashion with regards to policy, with government and parliament at the highest level and citizens, both individually and collectively, residing at the lowest.

I mean, this country is always like that, it has to be from top down. (23, PLHIV)

Those participants interviewed from the PLHIV and NGO community felt that they had little bargaining power in terms of influencing policy, and this is largely due to the structure of the organisation that represents them, the Malaysian Aids Council. The Malaysian Aids Council is the umbrella organisation which represents the various HIV NGOs within Malaysia and is considered to be independent of the government. Despite this, up to half of the finances which are received by the Malaysian Aids Council come directly from the Malaysian government, which makes the notion of their independence somewhat questionable.

Regardless of how funds are generated, they are then distributed by the Malaysian Aids Council to the myriad of HIV NGOs, each with their individual focus. Some of the smaller and newer HIV NGOs focus on support for children living with HIV, or housewives who were infected from their husbands who are now living with HIV. There are also organisations such as the PT Foundation that caters to all but works in particular with the marginalised of society, the transgender community, MSM and sex workers. With this in mind, one wonders whether there may be some pressure, even in its most subtle of forms, for the Council to distribute resources to the more socially appealing HIV NGOs.

Among the interviewees, there were differing thoughts regarding whether the Council was independent of government or not, with one participant from the Council arguing that the fact that they work so closely with government is an enabler as they were able to influence policy making decision indirectly. Another participant from the Council strongly felt that receiving funding and working so closely with the government resulted in an unavoidable conflict of interest at best, whilst it hindered the ability of PLHIV groups to voice their opinions, act and be critical of the government because doing so might result in harmful consequences, for example funding cuts. The Malaysian Aids Council was also under pressure from the general public as citizens who can raise matters in parliament, hence the belief that a bottom-up influence can also be exerted and why MAC is keen to engage with the general public, often with religious leaders as gatekeepers of the community.

This raises the question as to whether the general public as citizens are essentially silent stakeholders or at least influencers of a sort. In any case, a bottom-up change to policy as resulted from the Treatment Action Campaign in reducing the price of antiretrovirals in South Africa requires a strong civil society (Barmania and Lister 2013), which may not be feasible in Malaysia. Thus, it is evident that the perception was that the arbiters of power in HIV prevention policy were the Ministry of Health and the religious leaders, under the auspice of the governmental Department of Religious Affairs. People living with HIV felt that they had no real power or significant influence over policy, whereas outside international organisations, such as the United Nations, had that potential.

Stakeholder Understanding of HIV Transmission and Prevention

Amongst participants who responded to the questionnaire, there was relatively good knowledge of how HIV was transmitted. There was a sense from interviews that attitudes towards people with HIV had changed and softened over time, but that there was still a great degree of stigma, discrimination and moral and religious judgement associated with HIV infection.

With regards to correct knowledge of HIV transmission, from the surveys it was evident that the distribution of those who correctly answered questions about differed across the three main stakeholders, as one might expect. The Ministry of Health scored highest, with PLHIV following and the religious leaders scoring lowest.

Upon further testing it was clear that the difference in distribution of correct knowledge of HIV transmission across stakeholders was statistically significant. There were differences to scores of correct knowledge of HIV transmission when looked at specifically in relation to education level; those having had an advanced tertiary level education scored higher than those who had only primary level education. PLHIV scored relatively well for correct knowledge of HIV transmission, lower than the Ministry of Health but higher than religious leaders. However, it is worth noting that in the interviews many participants who were living with HIV said that before their diagnosis they themselves knew little about HIV transmission, as exemplified by the excerpt below:

> Before she got positive, she never knew what is HIV, how you get it; she only knew that how to use a condom. (6, PLHIV Transgender Woman)

Religious leaders scored lowest amongst all the stakeholder groups for correct knowledge of HIV transmission, which was also expected but highlights an area which could definitely be improved. When analysing the responses, looking at HIV transmission knowledge, there were certain questions on which religious leaders consistently scored lowest. For example, in respect of correct knowledge of HIV transmission through insect bites, religious leaders scored lowest at only 59%, whilst PLHIV scored 87% and individuals in the Ministry of Health 93%. This indicates an area where religious leaders need some assistance in increasing their overall knowledge of HIV transmission; a good mechanism would be increased engagement with JAKIM, who are already working on educating religious leaders. When asked what the causes of HIV were during an interview, one religious leader saying:

> HIV is spread from sexual act or injection. That's the only two ways; there is no more ways.
> (12, Religious Leader)

There were differences as to where various stakeholders acquired their general knowledge of HIV, with the Ministry of Health favouring their own sources and health care workers, religious leaders favouring television, and PLHIV favouring the internet. This also corresponded with some of the information regarding resources for HIV knowledge quoted in the interviews, with many PLHIV saying that information was acquired through the internet, social media and informal networks of friends, suggesting that peer education and provision of information sources accessible online would be beneficial:

> So from the internet, they get the information from there. (19, PLHIV)

These findings are consistent with other scholars such as Jahanfar et al. (2010), who found that the main source of knowledge of HIV amongst Malaysian university students was through the internet. It is well known that the internet is increasingly used for sex education (e.g. Simon and Daneback 2013).

With regards to knowledge of HIV prevention, there again was a statistically significant difference in the distribution of correct knowledge across the three groups of stakeholders. In addition, there were again differences with regards to education level, with those who had gone on to higher education scoring best.

It was interesting and perhaps unsurprising to note that there was a statistically significant difference in the proportions who correctly answered the question about whether HIV could be prevented through condom usage during sexual activity, with PLHIV scoring highest at 92%, the Ministry of Health lower at 89% and religious leaders the lowest at 77%.

Furthermore, there were differences across the three stakeholder groups in the approaches they felt should be taken to prevent HIV with PLHIV believing that better access to condoms, more of an enabling environment and better education and awareness around HIV were the best ways. Religious leaders felt that educating people about Islam was the best way of preventing HIV, which makes sense given that the promotion of Islam and Islamic values is one of their core functions.

Transgender Women and Men Who Have Sex with Men

Transgender Women

In Islamic teachings emulating the characteristics of the opposite gender of birth is not allowed and neither is changing one's gender. In fact, altering one's appearance is seen as not agreeing with the decree of Allah and challenging God. In Islamic scriptures men are expressly chastised for keeping their hair long or wearing silk, both of which are seen as acting in an effeminate way.

In the interviews there was acknowledgement of medical cases of individuals born with ambiguous genitalia, known as *khunsa*. Such cases were rare and mostly not applicable to the transgender community in Malaysia. In the interviews, even in the case of medically confirmed cases of *khunsa*, it was mentioned that either the individual or parents of the individual would have to choose the most appropriate gender based on both physical and psychological characteristics; there was no acceptance of a third gender.

Undertaking HIV prevention activities that target transgender groups is thus made exceedingly difficult for a number of reasons. The Islamic rulings on transgenderism affect public perception of the transgender community, marginalising them from the mainstream Malaysian community and creating more stigma and discrimination. This leads to difficulty in accessing the transgender community to provide HIV prevention services as they become harder to reach as they move underground.

Transgender women in Malaysia may have reservations about accessing health services (KRYSS 2012) as they are hesitant about the reception they will receive from health professionals, being concerned whether they will be classified as 'male' or 'female' in any documentation. As one transgender participant put it:

> I don't know what to put, female or male; sometimes they still discriminate us. Doctor OK, I don't trust with nurse, doctor yes, but nurse no, they [nurses] some of them are really bad mouthed, bad service. (5, Transgender Woman)

This can hinder a transgender person's willingness to access services. Some of the transgender women interviewed had first-hand negative experiences with health care workers, who were seen as untrustworthy and unprofessional; this meant transgender women would be less likely to access services from mainstream health care providers.

Furthermore, as some transgender women are engaged in sex work, those in the transgender women community are now frequently assumed to be sex workers, which is stigmatising, incorrect and makes HIV prevention more difficult.

Some Islamic religious leaders, such as JAKIM, make a genuine attempt to reach out to transgender communities; they understand that transgender people exist in Malaysia but wish to keep them under 'control'. Under the 'HIV and Islam' programme, religious leaders invite those from the transgender community to attend the voluntary *muhayam* camp, which JAKIM claims is a spiritual retreat intended to increase their faith not to convert them back to their original gender.

However, the transgender community takes a differing view and labels these retreats as 'conversion camps', and there is growing distrust and tension between the transgender community and religious leaders. The camps were seen by the transgender community as being highly offensive to them as the camps' existence failed to acknowledge the fundamental belief of those in the transgender community that their gender is not a feature that can be changed back or forth, like a lifestyle choice, but is an essential part of their identity.

Furthermore, Islamic rulings on transgenderism and sex work are imbedded in the legal (Syariah 1997) system (a dual system, criminal and *Sharia*) which affects both the law itself and the regulation of that law by the police and authorities. While it is not within the scope of this study to make judgements on the laws of Malaysia, especially referring to those that relate to sexual conduct and whether they should or should not be decriminalised, legalised or remain intact, we do wish to highlight the possible influence of Islamic rulings on the environment faced by individuals who are at risk of HIV infection and subsequent development of poor health.

During the course of the interviews PLHIV mentioned that the current legal system does not create an enabling environment for HIV prevention services for transgender women. These findings are consistent with research undertaken by Human Rights Watch and documentation from a review of the legal environment for HIV prevention in Malaysia relating to transgender women and MSM (HRW 2014; UN 2014).

A number of transgender participants said that they had experienced discrimination and victimisation by the police. This is a highly contentious issue whereby some groups feel that the occurrence of police discrimination and victimisation has been greatly exaggerated by outside human rights organisations, such as Human Rights Watch and other NGOs, whilst other groups believe it has not been acknowledged at all. Nevertheless, during the course of this study it was suggested that the transgender community was more vulnerable to corruption and extortion from the police, especially when carrying condoms for use in HIV prevention whether in their private lives or when working as a sex worker.

In the interviews, a few participants across stakeholder groups considered trans-gender women to be less well educated and thus more susceptible to police extor-tion. From the quantitative component of the study, the education level of the transgender women was lowest of all the genders. In any case, regardless of the reasoning, the transgender community felt more comfortable and 'safe' approach-ing and interacting with NGOs in relation to HIV prevention services. Such NGOs (like the PT Foundation) are at an advantage as they have members of the transgen-der and sex worker community within them and this provides access and trust. These NGOs can capitalise on this to provide services which people feel safe using. Unfortunately, such organisations often receive inadequate funding, and find it dif-ficult to continue to operate and provide such services; this represents a lost oppor-tunity, by not capitalising on the one group that has extensive access to the most marginalised of groups.

Thus, Islamic rulings on transgenderism either directly or indirectly create a challenge as they create a difficult climate within which to undertake HIV preven-tion services.

Men Who Have Sex with Men

In Islamic teachings the act of men having sex with men is explicitly mentioned in the *Qu'ran* and strictly forbidden; however, the idea of 'homosexuality' or 'sexual orientation' are Western concepts (Halstead and Reiss 2003) that were never specifi-cally mentioned. This is because there is a demarcation between the sexual 'act' and orientation, whereby it is the sexual act that is considered haram; i.e. whether a man acts on his orientation or not by engaging in anal or oral sex with another man is not relevant, the act is still *haram*. The concept of being 'gay' is not really one that many men who have sex with men in Malaysia identify with or relate to.

The *Qur'an* cites the story of *Lut* as strong condemnation for MSM, with the historical town finally being destroyed after the men in it engaged in such prolific an inappropriate sexual activity. Societal attitudes in Malaysia to MSM are scathing and acquiring HIV was widely seen as a punishment for being gay.

Those who are MSM are well aware of both Islamic teaching and the widespread condemnation of their actions by Malaysian society, which creates a lot of stigma directed towards them. In addition, there are also feelings of shame and self-stigmatisation and difficulties in reconciling being MSM with the knowledge that such actions are considered haram. As a result, MSM activities are drawn under-ground, with many from the MSM group feeling social and religious pressure to get married to a woman regardless of whether they wish to or not. This poses a myriad of other problems, such as furthering the HIV epidemic and making access to such men difficult.

Different stakeholders have varying experiences of and effectiveness at access-ing those who are MSM. Those organisations that do have good access to MSM tend to be NGOs which have MSM members. Normally, the main approach to HIV prevention amongst MSM would be distribution of condoms and lubricants but whilst the MOH distributes condoms it does not distribute lubricants. In addition, carrying condoms can be used, theoretically, as circumstantial evidence. Islamic teachings inspire to a degree the legal environment in Malaysia, whereby a man who has sex with a man can be charged with committing sodomy under section 377 of the penal code. Although very few have actually been charged with sodomy in Malaysia, simply the fear of knowing such a law exists creates fear and stigma amongst the MSM community.

This all serves to increase the challenging nature of providing services to MSM groups, by driving the epidemic and such individuals underground, creating difficulties for them to access services and be accessed. It also increases reluctance to be tested for HIV, ultimately creating a challenging environment in which to provide HIV prevention services.

The Consequences of Islamic Rulings on Sex Outside Marriage

Islamic rulings are clear that sex outside the confines of marriage is forbidden (*haram*); therefore, premarital and extramarital sexual activity are not permissible, as well as same-sex sexual relations or any form of sex work. Such activities are against the teachings of Islam and are seen to be damaging on multiple levels, to the individual, family and society as well as the Muslim *ummah*. Notwithstanding this, people often do not act in accordance with the teachings prescribed in the *Qu'ran* and Sunnah. This often results in a culture of denial and silence and presents a major issue when society is confronted with issues such as HIV. Firstly, how does one have public health interventions relating to HIV when your core belief is that there should not be a need for such interventions in the first place, since if society was living in accordance with Islam no one should become infected with HIV, a sentiment expressed by a number of religious leaders interviewed? Secondly, how does one tackle HIV prevention to minimise the risk to those who are engaging in sexual activity outside marriage, whilst also not encouraging the practice to others, or being seen to endorse it? It constitutes a very difficult balancing act whereby one has to take into consideration protecting the Islamic code of sexual conduct in Malaysia whilst protecting the health of those who are at risk from HIV.

Young Malaysians are taught about sex before they embark on marriage, within the compulsory premarital counselling course. Sex education in schools and universities is not considered in keeping with Islamic principles, so for the majority it is often not included in teaching or, if it is, is limited to human reproduction. There is certainly little mention of how to negotiate sex or protect yourself from HIV by using condoms, as is common in so-called comprehensive sex education programmes in many other parts of the world (e.g. Advocates for Youth 2009).

In Islamic doctrine there is not a specific ruling on condoms; however, the opinion amongst religious leaders in Malaysia is that their use is permissible only for married couples as contraception or in the case of serodiscordant couples. Whilst some viewed condoms as a neutral tool, other stakeholders believed that their use would encourage promiscuity and sex outside marriage and thus their distribution was categorically against the stance of most religious leaders, including JAKIM. In the surveys it was evident that religious leaders were less likely to see condom use as a method to prevent HIV compared with PLHIV (who were most positive about them) and the Ministry of Health.

For those working with MSM, transgender and sex worker groups, condoms were the mainstay of their HIV prevention mode, yet they were working in a climate where the use of condoms was looked upon with suspicion, which created a culture of not using condoms at all. This had implications for the wider society as those who frequented and used the services of sex worker were less likely to request the use of a condom and sex workers were often ill equipped to negotiate their use. Furthermore, there was a fear of even carrying a condom as it was perceived that this could be used as incriminating evidence by police or enforcement agencies, thus creating another barrier to their usage.

A premarital HIV screening test is compulsory for Muslims before they can proceed to marriage, but is not required for non-Muslims. In fact, the inception and implementation of the pre-marital HIV test is an interesting demonstration of the process of how strategies that intersect health and religion are undertaken as well as of the close ties between the Ministry of Health and religious leaders. It also highlights the importance of the use of language in HIV prevention policies, with the premarital test deemed as voluntary under the auspices of the Ministry of Health but mandatory through the Department of Religious Affairs. Language was also used in attempts to induce public acceptability as well as be diplomatic; however, it was still evident that there were underlying tensions between stakeholders.

Health policies do not exist in a vacuum but are set within a socio-political context affected by both national and international interests. In Malaysia, Islam is embedded within the constitution, which goes back historically to when Malaysia was granted independence after being incorporated into the British Empire. With this in mind, it is understandable that some stakeholders may have a fear of new interventions and policies, for example, the commonly held view that sex education is designed to promote a Western agenda and morality, as described by one of the religious leaders:

> People think this is western agenda to talk about sex education ... to propagate free sex. (8, Religious Leader)

Ultimately, HIV prevention in a predominantly Muslim country is a difficult terrain to navigate and although great gains have been made, challenges undoubtedly remain. Some of the issues raised from this study relate to the central problem of how a Muslim country like Malaysia can and should respond in terms of HIV prevention. This is consistent with much of the literature relating to other countries forced to formulate strategies to deal with the increased prevalence of HIV, against a backdrop of a predominantly Muslim society, which may often oppose certain strategies on religious grounds. This has been the case in Muslim-predominant countries such as Iran (Razzaghi et al. 2006), and elsewhere in the Middle East and North Africa (Mumtaz et al. 2014), which have had to recognise and respond to HIV epidemics amongst high risk groups, such as Men who have Sex with Men. Hasnain (2005), in her analysis of the cultural approaches to harm reduction in Muslim countries, highlighted the fact that it was often the case that in Muslim countries, when faced with tackling HIV prevention, policy makers would chose to respond with a 'propagation of Muslim ideals', avoidance of sexual activity outside marriage, for example. As HIV can be transmitted through a range of activities, including sexual intercourse outside of marriage, which is forbidden in Islam, HIV becomes a moral issue and not just a public health one (Kelley and Eberstadt 2005).

Overall, Malaysia has been forward thinking and practical and has successfully implemented needle exchange programmes to counter the transmission of HIV through intravenous drug use (Shetty 2013; Barmania 2013), until recently the main driver of HIV. The purpose of this study has been to explore the role of Islam, more precisely, the perception of Islamic practices in shaping the health policies and strategies related to HIV prevention in Malaysia from the perspectives of selected stakeholders. There are certainly areas where the perception of Islamic practice makes HIV prevention difficult and others where it has been an asset that has been leveraged to promote better treatment and care for those living with HIV.

References

Advocates for Youth. (2009). *Comprehensive sex education: Research and results.* Washington DC: Advocates for Youth. Available at http://www.advocatesforyouth.org/storage/advfy/documents/fscse.pdf

Barmania, S. (2013). Malaysia makes progress against HIV, but challenges remain. *Lancet, 381,* 2070–2071.

Barmania, S., & Lister, G. (2013). Civil society organisations, global health governance and public diplomacy. In I. Kichbusch, G. Lister, M. Told, & N. Drager (Eds.), *Global health diplomacy: Concepts, issues, actors, instruments, fora and cases* (pp. 253–267). New York: Springer.

Halstead, J. M., & Reiss, M. J. (2003). *Values in sex education: From principles to practice.* London: RoutledgeFalmer.

Hasnain, M. (2005). Cultural approaches to HIV/AIDS harm reduction in Muslim countries. *Harm Reduction Journal, 2,* 23.

Human Rights Watch. (2014). *"I'm scared to be a woman" – Human rights abuses against transgender people in Malaysia.* New York: Human Rights Watch.

Islamic Education Trust Nigeria. (2015). *Shari'ah intelligence: The basic principles and objectives of Islamic Jurisprudence.* Kuala Lumpur: Interactive Dawah Training.

Jahanfar, S., Sann, L. M., & Rampal, L. (2010). Sexual behaviour, knowledge and attitudes of non-medical university students towards HIV/AIDS in Malaysia. *Shiraz E Medical Journal, 11*(3), 122–136.

Kelley, L. M., & Eberstadt, N. (2005). *Behind the veil of a public health crisis: HIV/AIDS in the Muslim world.* Washington: National Bureau of Asian Research.

KRYSS. (2012). *Violence: Through the lens of lesbians, bisexual women and transgender people in Asia.* Malaysia: On the record. New York: Outright Action International. https://www.out-rightinternational.org/content/violence-through-lens-lbt-people-asia

Mumtaz, G. R., Riedner, G., & Abu-Raddad, L. (2014). The emerging face of the HIV epidemic in the Middle East and North Africa. *Current Opinion in HIV and AIDS, 9,* 183–191.

Obermeyer, C. (2006). HIV in the Middle East. Prevalence of HIV in the Middle East is low but there is no room for complacency. *British Medical Journal, 333,* 851–854.

Razzaghi, E., Nassirimanesh, B., Afshar, P., Ohiri, K., Claeson, M., & Power, R. (2006). HIV/AIDS harm reduction in Iran. *Lancet, 368,* 434–435.

Shetty, P. (2013). Profile – Adeeba Kamarulzaman: Fighting HIV/AIDS in Malaysia. *Lancet, 381,* 2073.

Simon, L., & Daneback, K. (2013). Adolescents' use of the internet for sex education: A thematic and critical review of the literature. *International Journal of Sexual Health, 25*(4), 305–319.

Syariah. (1997). Laws of Malaysia Syariah criminal offences. Federal Territories Act 1997.

United Nations Malaysia. (2014). *The policy and legal environment related to HIV services in Malaysia – Review and consultation.* Kuala Lumpur: United Nations.

Chapter 6
Conclusions and Recommendations

Conclusions

The remit of this study is not to suggest whether laws should or should not be changed, engage in politics or undermine any stakeholder, but to look at the role of Islam in shaping HIV prevention policies in Malaysia in an academic, impartial fashion without judgement or patronising any viewpoint but with cultural and religious sensitivity. This study is the first of its kind to use primary data to endeavour to understand how Islam affects HIV prevention policy in Malaysia, a Muslim predominant population. Hitherto, there had been a dearth of information and this research aids in closing the gap of knowledge.

The study highlights the fact that Islam affects HIV prevention policy in Malaysia both directly and indirectly. The study demonstrates the extent to which Islam plays an influential role in shaping health policies and strategies related to HIV prevention in Malaysia. Furthermore, Islam affects not only the policies themselves but the process of their implementation, as well as the hierarchy of power amongst different stakeholder groups. Islam proved important for an understanding of issues concerned with health and wellbeing, sex outside marriage, transgender women and men who have sex with men. With regards to knowledge of HIV, the stakeholder groups differed in their knowledge of HIV transmission and prevention and the most common method for obtaining information about these was through the internet. Amongst the stakeholder groups, varying viewpoints are held as to what constitutes the right approach to HIV prevention in Malaysia. Often, the viewpoint of one stakeholder conflicts with that of another stakeholder, either directly or more subtly, as indicated in the language used by stakeholders. Nevertheless, there are also areas of broad consensus amongst the varying stakeholders, including the great onus of preventing harm in the Islamic tradition, which can be powerfully leveraged and utilised in HIV prevention strategies.

© The Author(s) 2018
S. Barmania, M.J. Reiss, *Islam and Health Policies Related
to HIV Prevention in Malaysia*, SpringerBriefs in Public Health,
https://doi.org/10.1007/978-3-319-68909-8_6

Recommendations

Change in Language

There needs to be a deliberate change in the language used, both in terms of written documentation and in spoken discussions, formally and informally, between and within stakeholder groups involved in HIV prevention in Malaysia. Some of the language in use, such as expressions like 'prostitution' or 'sodomy', contributes to existing stakeholder tensions, stigma and discrimination and implies moral and religious judgement. There should be a move away from such terms to more appropriate alternatives such as 'sex worker' and 'anal sex'. Appropriate language can promote dialogue and mutual respect and shift the conversation towards disease prevention rather than morality. Utilisation of words which place emphasis on 'disease prevention' will hopefully help to move the focus and change the paradigm to a more public health centric attitude.

Utilisation of Islamic Principles in HIV Prevention

There should be an emphasis on Islamic principles, such as compassion and being merciful, in the HIV response as well as reminders of the importance of health and preservation of human life in Islam. There should be renewed debate amongst stakeholders and specifically with Islamic scholars and religious leaders regarding principles that may or may not be appropriate in discussions relating to the HIV response. Concepts such as *maslaha*, what is in the public interest, *isthtihad* and greater and lesser harm (*darar*) are ideas that could be looked into more deeply. These principles could be taken up by the Ministry of Health as justification for certain HIV prevention measures, for example.

Redistribution of Power

There should be redistribution of power so that the PLHIV groups have more of an equal voice and influence in comparison with other stakeholders, such as the Ministry of Health, in terms of health policy and strategies related to HIV prevention. In addition, as the Malaysian Aids Council (MAC) is the umbrella body for all the PLHIV NGOs in Malaysia, there needs to be clarification of the MAC position in terms of independence from the government, given its funding links with the Ministry of Health. The MAC cannot truly be effective in advocating for the concerns of people living with HIV if it is not truly independent of government. This change in power dynamic to a less hierarchal model could be negotiated and overseen through the United Nations in Malaysia.

Dialogue

There should be meaningful dialogue between those stakeholders involved in HIV prevention, including the Ministry of Health, religious departments and PLHIV groups, including transgender, MSM and sex worker communities. The dialogue should specifically concentrate on understanding the issues and viewpoints of the other stakeholders to overcome some of the suspicion and distrust between stakeholders, so that they all parties are able to work more closely as a team, whilst also feeling comfortable enough to disagree respectfully.

Sex and Relationship Education in Education System

A comprehensive sex and relationship education (SRE) package should be implemented in schools and universities; such a package would include awareness about HIV/AIDS and HIV transmission and methods of prevention. The package would be culturally and religiously sensitive, with a focus on disease prevention and public health and in line with Islamic ideals, whilst also acknowledging reality. There needs to be extensive consultations with representatives of universities and schools as well as religious leaders, the Ministry of Health, the Ministry of Education and NGOs regarding what the curriculum would include, followed by a pilot with a view to rolling out the initiative in other areas of Kuala Lumpur. There should be a clear indication as to which body is responsible for the implementation of SRE—our recommendation is that the Ministry of Education is the most appropriate one—with fixed outputs as well as start and end dates. In addition, advice should be sought from other Muslim predominant countries that have been effective in implementing SRE within school settings.

Uploading Correct and Useful Information Through the Internet and Social Media

The internet and social media should be explored in more depth as conduits for disseminating information on the prevention of HIV. The internet is readily accessible in both urban and rural areas, gives privacy to those wishing to acquire information and avoids public condemnation and suspicion. Websites which target youths and young adults as well as high risk groups, such as MSM, transgender and sex worker communities, should be used to provide correct information regarding HIV transmission and prevention and where to access further confidential services from NGOs and governmental and private health sectors.

Greater NGO Support

There is need for greater support for organisations that work with high risks groups, such as the PT Foundation. These NGOs have long established access and networks deep within communities which have been and still are hard to reach, such as MSM, transgender and sex worker groups. There needs to be greater financial and pastoral support from the Ministry of Health and the MAC, including training of those within the MAC itself. NGOs are well placed within the community to provide peer education.

Ability to Opt Out

There needs to be a genuine appreciation and acknowledgment that as much as individuals may endeavour to be neutral and impartial, no one leaves their personal views behind entirely when in a professional capacity and that some individuals working in HIV feel conflicted, for example, with respect to the issue of distributing condoms. This is serious point because in western medicine there is generally the availability to 'opt out' of participating in certain practices. For example, in the UK, opting out is permitted under General Medical Council guidelines for personal, ethical or religious reasons, as in the case of not providing termination of pregnancy (but referring the patient to someone who does) without being seen to neglect professional duties. Such measures in themselves are not without controversy but they do allow an avenue for those medical doctors to contravene neither their professional duty nor their moral belief. It also may be better than having to keep up the very thinly veiled illusion of impartiality, when it is widely known that individuals completely disagree with such actions. Thus, having the option for those within any organisations (for example the Ministry of Health) to opt out or be transferred to a different department and be replaced with someone who has less of a personal objection (a non-Muslim counterpart, perhaps) may provide a better and more comfortable working environment for all stakeholders.

Utilisation of Religious Leaders

Religious leaders should be commended for some of the work that they have done, such as provision of Islamic burial services for those who have died from AIDS, and be utilised as an entry point within communities to disseminate correct information about HIV, perhaps during the Friday *khutbahs*. In addition, religious leaders can play an important role in mitigating the stigma and discrimination faced by those living with HIV as well as providing information and referring to NGOs.

Greater Emphasis of Condom Usage

There should be a greater emphasis placed on condom usage as a tool for HIV prevention amongst high risk communities, such as transgender individuals, sex workers and MSM. This should be set against a culturally appropriate back drop with understanding of the Muslim context. In addition, there needs to be purchasing of both condoms and lubricants by the Ministry of Health which can then be distributed by NGOs, health facilities and other groups and those that feel comfortable doing so, a referral process of sorts.

Increased Public Awareness of HIV

There needs to be a greater awareness of HIV in Malaysia in general, the extent of the problem, the ways in which it is transmitted and how it can be prevented. This should be circulated through newspapers, television and radio in a non-judgemental manner.

Peer Education

A greater emphasis should be placed on peer-to-peer education for issues relating to HIV. Honest discussions, whereby those infected with HIV or affected by HIV can be invited to participating schools and universities to share their stories of living with HIV, should be encouraged.

Greater Transparency

There should be greater transparency in terms of funding arrangements and potential conflicts of interests for all stakeholders. For example, there should be clearer procedures as to why some HIV NGOs receive funding while others do not, or are discontinued. Transparent guidelines should be produced, outlining what position certain stakeholders have, and what is and is not within their remit.

Further Research

Finally, there needs to be more research, focussing on the influence of Islam in particular and religion in general on health and perceptions of health. Further research, both in Malaysia and elsewhere, could focus on the myriad of ways that Islam affects health, including mental and dietary health. In the context of HIV in Malaysia, comparable research to that reported here should be undertaken outside the Klang valley, in less urban and more rural areas, where religious leaders may have greater impact. It would be valuable to expand the geographical area internationally, collecting primary data from key stakeholders and analysing the role of Islam in HIV prevention policies in other Muslim countries.

Overall, this study has highlighted the fact that the interrelationships between Islam and health are surprisingly little charted, but wait to be researched. However, such research will not be possible without the funding required to conduct it.

Index

A
Abstinence, Be faithful and Condom' (ABC) campaigns, 2
Access, HIV services, 19, 20
Acquired Immune Deficiency Syndrome (AIDS), 3
Asia Pacific Coalition on Male (APCOM) sexual health, 12
Association of South East Asian countries (ASEAN), 7

C
Condoms
  distribution, 44, 45
  forbidden in Islam, 47
  haram, 48
  HIV prevention, 48
  JAKIM, 47
  pregnancy, 49
  promotion, 20, 21
  sex outside marriage, 47
  usage, 47–49

D
Dialogue, 89

E
Emphasis of condom usage, 91

F
Faith-based organisations (FBOs), 2, 3
Female sex workers, 13
Free sex, 67

G
Global HIV epidemic, 8–10

H
Harm reduction, 16, 17
High risk group, 10
HIV knowledge, 37–40
HIV prevention, 43–47
HIV prevention policy, 87
HIV/AIDS epidemic, 10
Human immunodeficiency virus (HIV)
  awareness and utilization, 19
  denial, stigma and discrimination, 37
  diagnosis, 39
  female sex workers, 13
  Islamic engagement, 18, 19
  knowledge and perceptions, 15, 16
  Muslim World, 3–4
  prevention, 38
  public awareness, 91
  religion, 3
  stigma and discrimination, 21
  testing, 20
  transgender women, 14, 15
Human rights, 57, 58

© The Author(s) 2018
S. Barmania, M.J. Reiss, *Islam and Health Policies Related to HIV Prevention in Malaysia*, SpringerBriefs in Public Health, https://doi.org/10.1007/978-3-319-68909-8

Printed in the United States
By Bookmasters